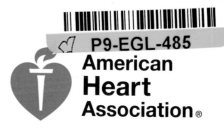

American
Heart
Association®

life is why™

ADVANCED CARDIOVASCULAR LIFE SUPPORT

PROVIDER MANUAL

ISBN 978-1-61669-400-5
Printed in the United States of America

First American Heart Association Printing March 2016
10 9 8 7 6 5 4 3 2

Acknowledgments

The American Heart Association thanks the following people for their contributions to the development of this manual: Michael W. Donnino, MD; Kenneth Navarro, MEd, LP; Katherine Berg, MD; Steven C. Brooks, MD, MHSc; Julie Crider, PhD; Mary Fran Hazinski, RN, MSN; Theresa A. Hoadley, RN, PhD, TNS; Sallie Johnson, PharmD, BCPS; Venu Menon, MD; Susan Morris, RN; Peter D. Panagos, MD; Michael Shuster, MD; David Slattery, MD; and the AHA ACLS Project Team.

 To find out about any updates or corrections to this text, visit **www.heart.org/cpr**, navigate to the page for this course, and click on "Updates."

To access the Student Website for this course, go to **www.heart.org/eccstudent** and enter this code: acls15

Contents

Contents

Part 5
The ACLS Cases   43

Contents

Contents

Contents

Contents

Appendix   155

Index   179

Note on Medication Doses

Emergency cardiovascular care is a dynamic science. Advances in treatment and drug therapies occur rapidly. Readers should use the following sources to check for changes in recommended doses, indications, and contraindications: the ECC Handbook, available as optional supplementary material, and the package insert product information sheet for each drug and medical device.

Contents

life is why.™

At the American Heart Association, we want people to experience more of life's precious moments. That's why we've made better heart and brain health our mission. It's also why we remain committed to exceptional training—the act of bringing resuscitation science to life—through genuine partnership with you. Only through our continued collaboration and dedication can we truly make a difference and save lives.

Until there's a world free of heart disease and stroke, the American Heart Association will be there, working with you to make a healthier, longer life possible for everyone.

Why do we do what we do?
life is why.

Life Is Why is a celebration of life. A simple yet powerful answer to the question of why we should all be healthy in heart and mind. It also explains why we do what we do: Lifesaving work. Every day.

Throughout your student manual, you will find information that correlates what you are learning in this class to **Life Is Why** and the importance of cardiovascular care. Look for the **Life Is Why** icon (shown at right), and remember that what you are learning today has an impact on the mission of the American Heart Association.

We encourage you to discover your **Why** and share it with others. Ask yourself, what are the moments, people, and experiences I live for? What brings me joy, wonder, and happiness? Why am I partnering with the AHA to help save lives? Why is cardiovascular care important to me? The answer to these questions is your **Why.**

Instructions

Please find on the back of this page a chance for you to participate in the AHA's mission and **Life Is Why** campaign. Complete this activity by filling in the blank with the word that describes your **Why.**

Share your "_____ **Is Why**" with the people you love, and ask them to discover their **Why.**

Talk about it. Share it. Post it. Live it.   #lifeiswhy   #CPRSavesLives

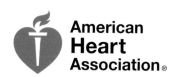

   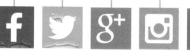

is why.

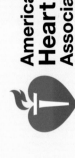

American
Heart
Association®

life is why™

Part 1

Introduction

Course Description and Goal

The Advanced Cardiovascular Life Support (ACLS) Provider Course is designed for healthcare providers who either direct or participate in the management of cardiopulmonary arrest or other cardiovascular emergencies. Through didactic instruction and active participation in simulated cases, students will enhance their skills in the recognition and intervention of cardiopulmonary arrest, immediate post–cardiac arrest, acute arrhythmia, stroke, and acute coronary syndromes (ACS).

The goal of the ACLS Provider Course is to improve outcomes for adult patients of cardiac arrest and other cardiopulmonary emergencies through early recognition and interventions by high-performance teams.

Course Objectives

Upon successful completion of this course, students should be able to

- Apply the Basic Life Support (BLS), Primary, and Secondary Assessment sequences for a systematic evaluation of adult patients
- Perform prompt, high-quality BLS, including prioritizing early chest compressions and integrating early automated external defibrillator (AED) use
- Recognize respiratory arrest
- Perform early management of respiratory arrest
- Discuss early recognition and management of ACS, including appropriate disposition
- Discuss early recognition and management of stroke, including appropriate disposition
- Recognize bradyarrhythmias and tachyarrhythmias that may result in cardiac arrest or complicate resuscitation outcome
- Perform early management of bradyarrhythmias and tachyarrhythmias that may result in cardiac arrest or complicate resuscitation outcome
- Recognize cardiac arrest
- Perform early management of cardiac arrest until termination of resuscitation or transfer of care, including immediate post–cardiac arrest care
- Evaluate resuscitative efforts during a cardiac arrest through continuous assessment of cardiopulmonary resuscitation (CPR) quality, monitoring the patient's physiologic response, and delivering real-time feedback to the team
- Model effective communication as a member or leader of a high-performance team
- Recognize the impact of team dynamics on overall team performance

- Discuss how the use of a rapid response team or medical emergency team may improve patient outcomes
- Define systems of care

Course Design

To help you achieve these objectives, the ACLS Provider Course includes practice learning stations and a Megacode evaluation station.

The *practice learning stations* give you an opportunity to actively participate in a variety of learning activities, including

- Simulated clinical scenarios
- Demonstrations by instructors or video
- Discussion and role playing
- Practice in effective high-performance team behaviors

In these learning stations, you will practice essential skills both individually and as part of a high-performance team. This course emphasizes effective team skills as a vital part of the resuscitative effort. You will have the opportunity to practice as a member and as a leader of a high-performance team.

At the end of the course, you will participate in a *Megacode evaluation station* to validate your achievement of the course objectives. A simulated cardiac arrest scenario will evaluate the following:

- Knowledge of core case material and skills
- Knowledge of algorithms
- Understanding of arrhythmia interpretation
- Use of appropriate basic ACLS drug therapy
- Performance as an effective leader of a high-performance team

Course Prerequisites and Preparation

The American Heart Association (AHA) limits enrollment in the ACLS Provider Course to healthcare providers who direct or participate in the resuscitation of a patient either in or out of hospital. Participants who enter the course must have the basic knowledge and skills to participate actively with the instructor and other students.

 Before the course, please read the *ACLS Provider Manual,* complete the mandatory Precourse Self-Assessment modules on the Student Website (**www.heart.org/eccstudent**), identify any gaps in your knowledge, and remediate those gaps by studying the applicable content in the *ACLS Provider Manual* or other supplementary resources, including the Student Website. A passing score for the self-assessment is 70%, and you may take it an unlimited number of times to achieve a passing score. **You will need to bring your Precourse Self-Assessment certificate with you to class.**

The following knowledge and skills are required for successful course completion:

- BLS skills
- Electrocardiogram (ECG) rhythm interpretation for core ACLS rhythms
- Knowledge of airway management and adjuncts
- Basic ACLS drug and pharmacology knowledge
- Practical application of ACLS rhythms and drugs
- Effective high-performance team skills

BLS Skills

The foundation of advanced life support is strong BLS skills. You must pass the high-quality BLS Testing Station to complete the ACLS course. *Make sure that you are proficient in BLS skills before attending the course.*

 Watch the High-Quality BLS Skills video found on the Student Website (**www.heart.org/eccstudent**). Review the High-Quality BLS Skills Testing Checklist located in the Appendix..

ECG Rhythm Interpretation for Core ACLS Rhythms

The basic cardiac arrest and periarrest algorithms require students to recognize these ECG rhythms:

- Sinus rhythm
- Atrial fibrillation and flutter
- Bradycardia
- Tachycardia
- Atrioventricular (AV) block
- Asystole
- Pulseless electrical activity (PEA)
- Ventricular tachycardia (VT)
- Ventricular fibrillation (VF)

 You will need to complete the ACLS Precourse Self-Assessment, which contains ECG rhythm identification, on the Student Website (**www.heart.org/eccstudent**). At the end of the assessment, you will receive your score and feedback to help you identify areas of strength and weakness. Remediate any gaps in your knowledge before entering the course. During the course, you must be able to identify and interpret rhythms during practice as well as during the final Megacode evaluation station.

Basic ACLS Drug and Pharmacology Knowledge

You must know the drugs and doses used in the ACLS algorithms. You will also need to know *when* to use *which* drug based on the clinical situation.

 You will need to complete the ACLS Precourse Self-Assessment, which contains pharmacology questions, on the Student Website (**www.heart.org/eccstudent**). At the end of the assessment, you will receive your score and feedback to help you identify areas of strength and weakness. Remediate any gaps in your knowledge before entering the course.

Course Materials

Course materials consist of the *ACLS Provider Manual,* Student Website (**www.heart.org/eccstudent**), 2 Pocket Reference Cards, and Precourse Preparation Checklist. The icon on the left directs you to additional supplementary information on the Student Website.

ACLS Provider Manual

The *ACLS Provider Manual* contains the basic information you need for effective participation in the course. This important material includes the systematic approach to a cardiopulmonary emergency, effective high-performance team communication, and the ACLS cases and algorithms. ***Please review this manual before attending the course. Bring it with you for use and reference during the course.***

The manual is organized into the following parts:

Part 1	Introduction
Part 2	Systems of Care
Part 3	Effective High-Performance Team Dynamics
Part 4	The Systematic Approach
Part 5	The ACLS Cases
Appendix	Testing Checklists and Learning Station Checklists
ACLS Pharmacology Summary Table	Basic ACLS drugs, doses, indications and contraindications, and side effects
2015 Science Summary Table	Highlights of 2015 science changes in the ACLS Provider Course
Glossary	Alphabetical list of terms and their definitions
Foundation Index	Pages where key subjects can be found (eg, epinephrine, cardioversion, pacing)
Index	

The AHA requires that students complete and pass the Precourse Self-Assessment found on the Student Website and print their scores for submission to their ACLS Instructor. The Precourse Self-Assessment allows students to understand gaps in knowledge required to participate in and pass the course. Supplementary topics located on the Student Website are useful but not essential for successful completion of the course.

Call-out Boxes

The *ACLS Provider Manual* contains important information presented in call-out boxes that require the reader's attention. Please pay particular attention to the call-out boxes, listed below:

Critical Concepts	Pay particular attention to the **Critical Concepts** boxes that appear in the *ACLS Provider Manual*. These boxes contain the most important information that you must know.
Caution	**Caution** boxes emphasize specific risks associated with interventions.
FYI 2015 Guidelines	**FYI 2015 Guidelines** boxes contain the new *2015 AHA Guidelines Update for CPR and Emergency Cardiovascular Care* (ECC) information.
Foundational Facts	**Foundational Facts** boxes contain basic information that will help you understand the topics covered in the course.
Life Is Why	**Life Is Why** boxes describe why taking this course matters.

Student Website

 The ACLS Student Website (**www.heart.org/eccstudent**) contains the following self-assessment and supplementary resources:

Resource	Description	How to Use
Mandatory Precourse Self-Assessment	The Precourse Self-Assessment evaluates a student's knowledge in 3 sections: rhythm, pharmacology, and practical application	Complete *before the course* to help evaluate your proficiency and determine the need for additional review and practice before the course

(continued)

(continued)

Resource	Description	How to Use
ACLS Supplementary Information	• Basic Airway Management • Advanced Airway Management • ACLS Core Rhythms • Defibrillation • Access for Medications • Acute Coronary Syndromes • Human, Ethical, and Legal Dimensions of ECC and ACLS • Web-Based Self-Assessment: Drugs Used in Algorithms	Additional information to supplement basic concepts presented in the ACLS course Some information is supplementary; other areas are for the interested student or advanced provider
High-Quality BLS video	• High-quality BLS • Compressions • Ventilations • AED use	
ACS video	• ST-segment elevation myocardial infarction (STEMI) • Chain of Survival • Supplementary oxygen • 12-lead ECG • Reperfusion • Percutaneous coronary intervention • Fibrinolytic therapy	
Stroke video	• Acute stroke • Chain of Survival • 8 D's of Stroke Care • Fibrinolytic therapy	
Airway Management video	• Airway adjuncts • Advanced airways • Confirmation devices	

Pocket Reference Cards

The Pocket Reference Cards are 2 stand-alone cards packaged with the *ACLS Provider Manual.* These cards can be carried in your pocket for quick reference on the following topics:

Topic	Reference Cards
Cardiac arrest, arrhythmias, and treatment	• Adult Cardiac Arrest Algorithms • Table with drugs and dosage reminders • Adult Immediate Post–Cardiac Arrest Care Algorithm • Adult Bradycardia With a Pulse Algorithm • Adult Tachycardia With a Pulse Algorithm
ACS and stroke	• Acute Coronary Syndromes Algorithm • Fibrinolytic Checklist for STEMI • Fibrinolytic Contraindications for STEMI • Adult Suspected Stroke Algorithm • Stroke Assessment—Cincinnati Prehospital Stroke Scale • Use of IV rtPA for Acute Ischemic Stroke • Hypertension Management in Acute Ischemic Stroke

Precourse Preparation Checklist

The Precourse Preparation Checklist is packaged with the *ACLS Provider Manual.* Please review and check the boxes after you have completed preparation for each section.

Requirements for Successful Course Completion

To successfully complete the ACLS Provider Course and obtain your course completion card, you must

- Pass the Adult High-Quality BLS Skills Test
- Pass the Bag-Mask Ventilation Skills Test, including oropharyngeal airway/nasopharyngeal airway insertion
- Demonstrate competency in learning station skills
- Pass the Megacode Test
- Pass the open-resource exam with a minimum score of 84%

Life Is Why

Saving Lives Is Why

Cardiac arrest remains a leading cause of death, so the AHA trains millions of people each year to help save lives both in and out of the hospital. This course is a key part of that effort.

ACLS Provider Manual Abbreviations

A	
ACE	Angiotensin-converting enzyme
ACLS	Advanced cardiovascular life support
ACS	Acute coronary syndromes
AED	Automated external defibrillator
AHF	Acute heart failure
AIVR	Accelerated idioventricular rhythm
AMI	Acute myocardial infarction
aPTT	Activated partial thromboplastin time
AV	Atrioventricular
B	
BLS	Basic life support: Check responsiveness, activate emergency response system, check carotid pulse, provide defibrillation
C	
CARES	Cardiac Arrest Registry to Enhance Survival
CCF	Chest compression fraction
CPR	Cardiopulmonary resuscitation
CPSS	Cincinnati Prehospital Stroke Scale
CQI	Continuous quality improvement
CT	Computed tomography
D	
DNAR	Do not attempt resuscitation
E	
ECG	Electrocardiogram
ED	Emergency department
EMS	Emergency medical services
ET	Endotracheal
F	
FDA	Food and Drug Administration
FIO_2	Fraction of inspired oxygen
G	
GI	Gastrointestinal

I	
ICU	Intensive care unit
INR	International normalized ratio
IO	Intraosseous
IV	Intravenous

L	
LV	Left ventricle or left ventricular

M	
mA	Milliamperes
MACE	Major adverse cardiac events
MET	Medical emergency team
MI	Myocardial infarction
mm Hg	Millimeters of mercury

N	
NIH	National Institutes of Health
NIHSS	National Institutes of Health Stroke Scale
NINDS	National Institute of Neurological Disorders and Stroke
NPA	Nasopharyngeal airway
NSAID	Nonsteroidal anti-inflammatory drug
NSTE-ACS	Non–ST-segment elevation acute coronary syndromes
NSTEMI	Non–ST-segment elevation myocardial infarction

O	
OPA	Oropharyngeal airway

P	
Paco$_2$	Partial pressure of carbon dioxide in arterial blood
PCI	Percutaneous coronary intervention
PE	Pulmonary embolism
PEA	Pulseless electrical activity
Petco$_2$	Partial pressure of end-tidal carbon dioxide
PT	Prothrombin time
pVT	Pulseless ventricular tachycardia

R	
ROSC	Return of spontaneous circulation
RRT	Rapid response team
rtPA	Recombinant tissue plasminogen activator
RV	Right ventricle or right ventricular

S	
SBP	Systolic blood pressure
STEMI	ST-segment elevation myocardial infarction
SVT	Supraventricular tachycardia
T	
TCP	Transcutaneous pacing
TTM	Targeted temperature management
U	
UA	Unstable angina
V	
VF	Ventricular fibrillation
VT	Ventricular tachycardia

Advanced Cardiovascular Life Support

ACLS providers face an important challenge—functioning as a team that implements and integrates both basic and advanced life support to save a person's life. The *2015 AHA Guidelines Update for CPR and ECC* reviewed evidence that shows that in both the in-hospital and out-of-hospital settings, many cardiac arrest patients do not receive high-quality CPR, and the majority do not survive. One study of in-hospital cardiac arrest showed that the quality of CPR was inconsistent and did not always meet guidelines recommendations.[1] Over the years, however, patient outcomes after cardiac arrest have improved. Table 1 shows the recent trends in survival in both out-of-hospital and in-hospital cardiac arrest in the United States.[2]

Table 1. Recent Cardiac Arrest Survival Data

Statistical Update	Out-of-Hospital Cardiac Arrest			In-Hospital Cardiac Arrest	
	Incidence, n	Bystander CPR (Overall), %	Survival Rate* (Overall), %	Incidence,[†] n	Survival Rate* (Adults), %
2015	326 200	45.9	10.6	209 000	25.5
2014	424 000	40.8	10.4	209 000	22.7
2013	359 400	40.1	9.5	209 000	23.9
2012	382 800	41.0	11.4	209 000	23.1
Baseline		31	7.9		19

*Survival to hospital discharge.

[†]Extrapolated incidence based on the same 2011 Get With The Guidelines-Resuscitation study.

To analyze these findings, a "back-to-basics" evidence review refocused on the essentials of CPR, the links in the Chain of Survival, and the integration of BLS with ACLS. Minimizing the interval between stopping chest compressions and delivering a shock (ie, minimizing the preshock pause) improves the chances of shock success[3] and patient survival.[4] Experts believe that high survival rates from both out-of-hospital and in-hospital sudden cardiac death are possible with strong systems of care.

High survival rates in studies are associated with several common elements:

- Training of knowledgeable healthcare providers
- Planned and practiced response
- Rapid recognition of sudden cardiac arrest
- Prompt provision of CPR
- Defibrillation as early as possible and within 3 to 5 minutes of collapse
- Organized post–cardiac arrest care

When trained persons implement these elements early, ACLS has the best chance of producing a successful outcome.

Critical Concepts

Optimization of ACLS

ACLS is optimized when a team leader effectively integrates high-quality CPR and minimal interruption of high-quality chest compressions with advanced life support strategies (eg, defibrillation, medications, advanced airway).

Critical Concepts

Minimize Interruptions in Compressions

Studies have shown that a reduction in the interval between stopping compressions and shock delivery can increase the predicted shock success. Interruptions in compressions should be limited to critical interventions (rhythm analysis, shock delivery, intubation, etc), and even then, these should be minimized to 10 seconds or less.

Closing the Gaps

Quality Assessment, Review, and Translational Science

Every emergency medical service (EMS) and hospital system should perform continuous quality improvement to assess its resuscitation interventions and outcomes through a defined process of data collection and review. There is now widespread consensus that the best way to improve either community or in-hospital survival from sudden cardiac arrest is to start with the standard "quality improvement model" and then modify that model according to the Chain of Survival metaphor. Each link in the chain comprises structural, process, and outcome variables that can be examined, measured, and recorded. System managers can quickly identify gaps that exist between observed processes and outcomes and local expectations or published "gold standards."

Life Is Why

Life Is Why

At the American Heart Association, we want people to experience more of life's precious moments. What you learn in this course can help build healthier, longer lives for everyone.

References

1. Abella BS, Alvarado JP, Myklebust H, et al. Quality of car-diopulmonary resuscitation during in-hospital cardiac arrest. *JAMA*. 2005;293(3):305-310.

2. Mozaffarian D, Benjamin EJ, Go AS, et al; on behalf of the American Heart Association Statistics Committee and Stroke Statistics Subcommittee. Heart disease and stroke statistics—2015 update: a report from the American Heart Association. *Circulation*. 2015;131(4):e29-e322.

3. Edelson DP, Abella BS, Kramer-Johansen J, et al. Effects of compression depth and pre-shock pauses predict defibrillation failure during cardiac arrest. *Resuscitation*. 2006;71(2):137-145.

4. Edelson DP, Litzinger B, Arora V, et al. Improving in-hospital cardiac arrest process and outcomes with performance debriefing. *Arch Intern Med*. 2008;168(10):1063-1069.

Part 2

Systems of Care

Introduction	A *system* is a group of regularly interacting and interdependent components. The system provides the links for the chain and determines the strength of each link and the chain as a whole. By definition, the system determines the ultimate outcome and provides collective support and organization. The ideal work flow to accomplish resuscitation successfully is highly dependent on the system of care as a whole.

Cardiopulmonary Resuscitation

Quality Improvement in Resuscitation Systems, Processes, and Outcomes	CPR is a series of lifesaving actions that improve the chance of survival after cardiac arrest. Although the optimal approach to CPR may vary, depending on the rescuer, the patient, and the available resources, the fundamental challenge remains how to achieve early and effective CPR.
A Systems Approach	In this part, we will focus on 2 distinct systems of care: the system for patients who arrest inside of the hospital and the one for those who arrest outside of it. We will set into context the building blocks for a system of care for cardiac arrest, with consideration of the setting, team, and available resources, as well as continuous quality improvement (CQI) from the moment the patient becomes unstable until after the patient is discharged.
	Healthcare delivery requires structure (eg, people, equipment, education) and process (eg, policies, protocols, procedures), which, when integrated, produce a system (eg, programs, organizations, cultures) leading to outcomes (eg, patient safety, quality, satisfaction). An effective system of care comprises all of these elements—structure, process, system, and patient outcomes—in a framework of CQI (Figure 1).

Taxonomy of Systems of Care: SPSO
Structure Process System Outcome

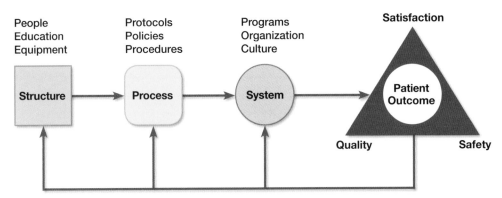

Figure 1. Taxonomy of systems of care.

Successful resuscitation after cardiac arrest requires an integrated set of coordinated actions represented by the links in the system-specific Chains of Survival (Figure 2).

Effective resuscitation requires an integrated response known as a *system of care*. Fundamental to a successful resuscitation system of care is the collective appreciation of the challenges and opportunities presented by the Chain of Survival. Thus, individuals and groups must work together, sharing ideas and information, to evaluate and improve their resuscitation system. Leadership and accountability are important components of this team approach.

To improve care, leaders must assess the performance of each system component. Only when performance is evaluated can participants in a system effectively intervene to improve care. This process of quality improvement consists of an iterative and continuous cycle of

- Systematic evaluation of resuscitation care and outcome
- Benchmarking with stakeholder feedback
- Strategic efforts to address identified deficiencies

While the care for all postresuscitation patients, regardless of where the arrest occurred, converges in the hospital, generally in an intensive care unit (ICU), the structure and process elements before that convergence vary highly for the 2 patient populations. Patients with out-of-hospital cardiac arrest (OHCA) depend on their community for support. Lay rescuers are expected to recognize a patient's distress, call for help, and initiate CPR and public-access defibrillation (PAD) until a team of professionally trained EMS providers assumes responsibility and transports the patient to an emergency department (ED) and/or cardiac catheterization lab before the patient is transferred to an ICU for continued care.

In contrast, patients with in-hospital cardiac arrest (IHCA) depend on a system of appropriate surveillance and prevention of cardiac arrest. When they do arrest, they depend on the smooth interaction of the institution's various departments and services and on a multidisciplinary team of professional providers, which includes physicians, nurses, respiratory therapists, pharmacists, counselors, and others.

IHCA

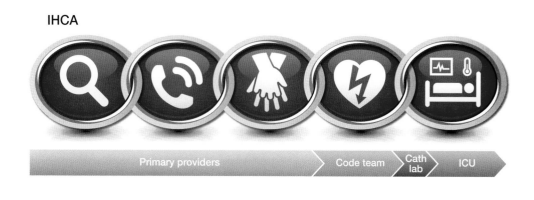

OHCA

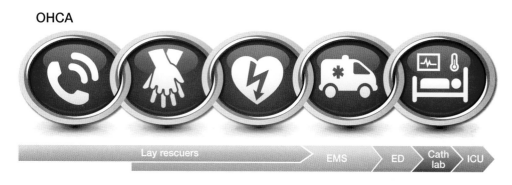

Figure 2. System-specific Chains of Survival.

Foundational Facts

Medical Emergency Teams and Rapid Response Teams

- Many hospitals have implemented the use of METs or RRTs. The purpose of these teams is to improve patient outcomes by identifying and treating early clinical deterioration (Figure 3). IHCA is commonly preceded by physiologic changes. In recent studies, nearly 80% of hospitalized patients with cardiorespiratory arrest had abnormal vital signs documented for up to 8 hours before the actual arrest. Many of these changes can be recognized by monitoring routine vital signs. Intervention before clinical deterioration or cardiac arrest may be possible.

- Consider this question: "Would you have done anything differently if you knew 15 minutes before the arrest that…?"

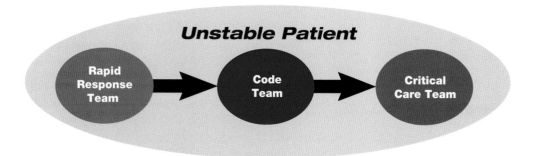

Figure 3. Management of life-threatening emergencies requires integration of multidisciplinary teams that can involve RRTs, cardiac arrest teams, and intensive care specialties to achieve survival of the patient. Team leaders have an essential role in coordination of care with team members and other specialists.

The classic resuscitation Chain of Survival concept linked the community to EMS and EMS to hospitals, with hospital care as the destination.[1] But patients with a cardiac emergency may enter the system of care at one of many different points (Figure 4).

They can present anywhere, anytime—on the street or at home, yes, but also in the hospital's ED, inpatient bed, ICU, operating suite, catheterization suite, or imaging department. The system of care must be able to manage cardiac emergencies wherever they occur.

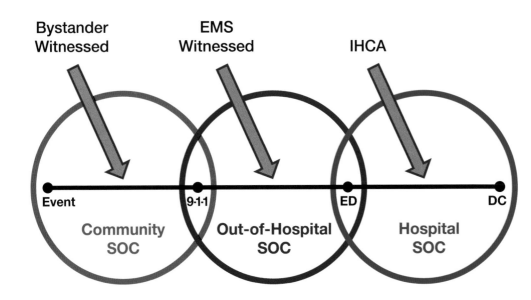

Figure 4. Patient's point of entry. Abbreviations: EMS, emergency medical services; IHCA, in-hospital cardiac arrest; SOC, system of care; DC, discharge.

Measurement

Continual efforts to improve resuscitation outcomes are impossible without data capture. The collection of resuscitation process measures is the underpinning of a system of care's quality improvement efforts. Quality improvement relies on valid assessment of resuscitation performance and outcome.

Utstein-style guidelines and templates have been prepared for reporting resuscitation outcomes after trauma and drowning.[2]

- The Utstein Guidelines[3] provide guidance for core performance measures, including
  - Rate of bystander CPR
  - Time to defibrillation
  - Time to advanced airway management
  - Time to first administration of resuscitation medication
  - Survival to hospital discharge

Monitors to measure CPR performance are now widely available.[4] They provide rescuers with invaluable real-time feedback on the quality of CPR delivered during resuscitative efforts, data for debriefing after resuscitation, and retrospective information for system-wide CPR CQI programs. Without CPR measurement and subsequent understanding of CPR performance, improvement and optimized performance cannot occur. Providing CPR without monitoring performance can be likened to flying an airplane without an altimeter.

Routinely available feedback on CPR performance characteristics includes chest compression rate, depth, and recoil.[4] Currently, certain important parameters (chest compression fraction and preshock, perishock, and postshock pauses) can be reviewed only retrospectively, whereas others (ventilation rate, airway pressure, tidal volume, and inflation duration) cannot be assessed adequately by current technology. Additionally, accelerometers are insensitive to mattress compression, and current devices often prioritize the order of feedback by use of a rigid algorithm in a manner that may not be optimal or realistic (eg, an accelerometer cannot measure depth if there is too much leaning, so the device will prioritize feedback to correct leaning before correcting depth). Although some software (automated algorithms) and hardware (smart backboard, dual accelerometers, reference markers, and others) solutions currently exist, continued development of optimal and widely available CPR monitoring is a key component to improved performance.

Life Is Why

High-Quality CPR Is Why

Early recognition and CPR are crucial for survival from cardiac arrest. By learning high-quality CPR, you'll have the ability to improve patient outcomes and save more lives.

Benchmarking and Feedback

Data should be systematically reviewed and compared internally to prior performance and externally to similar systems. Existing registries can facilitate this benchmarking effort. Examples include

- Cardiac Arrest Registry to Enhance Survival (CARES) for OHCA
- Get With The Guidelines®-Resuscitation program for IHCA

Change

Simply measuring and benchmarking care can positively influence outcome. However, ongoing review and interpretation are necessary to identify areas for improvement, such as

- Increased bystander CPR response rates
- Improved CPR performance
- Shortened time to defibrillation
- Citizen awareness
- Citizen and healthcare professional education and training

Summary

Over the past 50 years, the modern-era BLS fundamentals of early recognition and activation, early CPR, and early defibrillation have saved hundreds of thousands of lives around the world. However, we still have a long road to travel if we are to fulfill the potential offered by the Chain of Survival. Survival disparities presented a generation ago appear to persist. Fortunately, we currently possess the knowledge and tools—represented by the Chain of Survival—to address many of these care gaps, and future discoveries will offer opportunities to improve rates of survival.

Acute Coronary Syndromes

The primary goals of therapy for patients with acute coronary syndromes (ACS) are to

1. Reduce the amount of myocardial necrosis that occurs in patients with acute myocardial infarction, thus preserving left ventricular function, preventing heart failure, and limiting other cardiovascular complications

2. Prevent major adverse cardiac events: death, nonfatal myocardial infarction, and the need for urgent revascularization

3. Treat acute, life-threatening complications of ACS, such as ventricular fibrillation (VF), pulseless VT (pVT), unstable tachycardias, symptomatic bradycardias, pulmonary edema, cardiogenic shock, and mechanical complications of acute myocardial infarction

Starts "On the Phone" With Activation of EMS

Prompt diagnosis and treatment offers the greatest potential benefit for myocardial salvage. Thus, it is imperative that healthcare providers recognize patients with potential ACS to initiate evaluation, appropriate triage, and management as expeditiously as possible.

EMS Components

- Prehospital ECGs
- Notification of the receiving facility of a patient with possible ST-segment elevation myocardial infarction ("STEMI alert")
- Activation of the cardiac catheterization team to shorten reperfusion time
- Continuous review and quality improvement

Hospital-Based Components

- **ED protocols**
  - Activation of the cardiac catheterization laboratory
  - Admission to the coronary ICU
  - Quality assurance, real-time feedback, and healthcare provider education
- **Emergency physician**
  - Empowered to select the most appropriate reperfusion strategy
  - Empowered to activate the cardiac catheterization team as indicated
- **Hospital leadership**
  - Must be involved in the process and committed to support rapid access to STEMI reperfusion therapy

Acute Stroke

The healthcare system has achieved significant improvements in stroke care through integration of public education, emergency dispatch, prehospital detection and triage, hospital stroke system development, and stroke unit management. Not only have the rates of appropriate fibrinolytic therapy increased over the past 5 years, but overall stroke care has also improved, in part through the creation of stroke centers.

Regionalization of Stroke Care

With the National Institute of Neurological Disorders and Stroke recombinant tissue plasminogen activator (rtPA) trial,[5] the crucial need for local partnerships between academic medical centers and community hospitals became clear. The time-sensitive nature of stroke requires such an approach, even in densely populated metropolitan centers.

Community and Professional Education

Community and professional education is essential and has successfully increased the proportion of stroke patients treated with fibrinolytic therapy.

- Patient education efforts are most effective when the message is clear and succinct.
- Educational efforts need to couple the knowledge of the signs and symptoms of stroke with action—activate the emergency response system.

EMS

The integration of EMS into regional stroke models is crucial for improvement of patient outcomes.[6]

- EMS response personnel trained in stroke recognition
- Stroke-prepared hospitals–primary stroke centers
- Access to stroke expertise via telemedicine from the nearest stroke center

Post–Cardiac Arrest Care

The healthcare system should implement a comprehensive, structured, multidisciplinary system of care in a consistent manner for the treatment of post–cardiac arrest patients. Programs should address targeted temperature management (TTM), hemodynamic and ventilation optimization, immediate coronary reperfusion with percutaneous coronary intervention (PCI) for eligible patients, neurologic care and prognostication, and other structured interventions.

Patients who achieve return of spontaneous circulation (ROSC) after cardiac arrest in any setting have a complex combination of pathophysiologic processes described as post–cardiac arrest syndrome, which includes postarrest brain injury, postarrest myocardial dysfunction, systemic ischemia or reperfusion response, and persistent acute and chronic pathology that may have precipitated the cardiac arrest.[7] Post–cardiac arrest syndrome plays a significant role in patient mortality.

Individual hospitals with a high frequency of treating cardiac arrest patients show an increased likelihood of survival when these interventions are provided.[8,9]

Targeted Temperature Management

The *2015 AHA Guidelines Update for CPR and ECC* recommends that TTM interventions be administered to comatose (ie, lacking meaningful response to verbal commands) adult patients with ROSC after cardiac arrest, by selecting and maintaining a constant temperature between 32°C and 36°C (89.6°F and 95.2°F) for at least 24 hours.

Hemodynamic and Ventilation Optimization

Although providers often use 100% oxygen while performing the initial resuscitation, providers should titrate inspired oxygen during the post–cardiac arrest phase to the lowest level required to achieve an arterial oxygen saturation of 94% or greater, when feasible. This helps to avoid any potential complications associated with oxygen toxicity.

Avoid excessive ventilation of the patient because of potential adverse hemodynamic effects when intrathoracic pressures are increased and because of potential decreases in cerebral blood flow when partial pressure of carbon dioxide in arterial blood ($Paco_2$) decreases.

Healthcare providers may start ventilation rates at 10/min. Normocarbia (partial pressure of end-tidal carbon dioxide [$Petco_2$] of 30 to 40 mm Hg or $Paco_2$ of 35 to 45 mm Hg) may be a reasonable goal unless patient factors prompt more individualized treatment. Other $Paco_2$ targets may be tolerated for specific patients. For example, a higher $Paco_2$ may be permissible in patients with acute lung injury or high airway pressures. Likewise, mild hypocapnia might be useful as a temporary measure when treating cerebral edema, but hyperventilation could cause cerebral vasoconstriction. Providers should note that when a patient's temperature is below normal, laboratory values reported for $Paco_2$ might be higher than the actual values.

Healthcare providers should titrate fluid administration and vasoactive or inotropic agents as needed to optimize blood pressure, cardiac output, and systemic perfusion. The optimal post–cardiac arrest blood pressure remains unknown; however, a mean arterial pressure of 65 mm Hg or greater is a reasonable goal.

Immediate Coronary Reperfusion With PCI

After ROSC in patients in whom coronary artery occlusion is suspected, rescuers should transport the patient to a facility capable of reliably providing coronary reperfusion (eg, PCI) and other goal-directed post–cardiac arrest care therapies. The decision to perform PCI can be made irrespective of the presence of coma or the decision to induce hypothermia, because concurrent PCI and hypothermia are feasible and safe and have good outcomes.

Glycemic Control

Healthcare providers should not attempt to alter glucose concentration within a lower range (80 to 110 mg/dL [4.4 to 6.1 mmol/L]), because of the increased risk of hypoglycemia. The *2015 AHA Guidelines Update for CPR and ECC* does not recommend any specific target range of glucose management in adult patients with ROSC after cardiac arrest.

Neurologic Care and Prognostication

The goal of post–cardiac arrest management is to return patients to their prearrest functional level. Reliable early prognostication of neurologic outcome is an essential component of post–cardiac arrest care, but the optimal timing is important to consider. In patients treated with TTM, prognostication using clinical examination should be delayed until at least 72 hours after return to normothermia. For those not treated with TTM, the earliest time is 72 hours after cardiac arrest and potentially longer if the residual effect of sedation or paralysis confounds the clinical examination.

Education, Implementation, and Teams

The Chain of Survival is a metaphor used to organize and describe the integrated set of time-sensitive coordinated actions necessary to maximize survival from cardiac arrest. The use of evidence-based education and implementation strategies can optimize the links in the chain.

The Need for Teams

Mortality from IHCA remains high. The average survival rate is approximately 24%, despite significant advances in treatments. Survival rates are particularly poor for arrest associated with rhythms other than VF/pVT. Non-VF/pVT rhythms are present in more than 82% of arrests in the hospital.[10]

Many in-hospital arrests are preceded by easily recognizable physiologic changes, many of which are evident with routine monitoring of vital signs. In recent studies, nearly 80% of hospitalized patients with cardiorespiratory arrest had abnormal vital signs documented for up to 8 hours before the actual arrest. This finding suggests that there is a period of increasing instability before the arrest.

Cardiac Arrest Teams (In-Hospital)

Cardiac arrest teams are unlikely to prevent arrests because their focus has traditionally been to respond only after the arrest has occurred. Unfortunately, the mortality rate is more than 75% once the arrest occurs.[10]

Over the past few years, hospitals have expanded the focus to include patient safety and prevention of arrest. The best way to improve a patient's chance of survival from a cardiorespiratory arrest is to prevent it from happening.

Poor-quality CPR should be considered a preventable harm.[4] In healthcare environments, variability in clinician performance has affected the ability to reduce healthcare-associated complications,[11] and a standardized approach has been advocated to improve outcomes and reduce preventable harms.[12] Doing so requires a significant cultural shift within institutions. Actions and interventions need to be proactive with the goal of improving rates of morbidity and mortality rather than reacting to a catastrophic event.

Rapid assessment and intervention for many abnormal physiologic variables can decrease the number of arrests occurring in the hospital.

Rapid Response System

The wide variability in incidence and location of cardiac arrest in the hospital suggests potential areas for standardization of quality and prevention of at least some cardiac arrests. More than half of cardiac arrests in the hospital are the result of respiratory failure or hypovolemic shock, and the majority of these events are foreshadowed by changes in physiology, such as tachypnea, tachycardia, and hypotension. As such, cardiac arrest in the hospital often represents the progression of physiologic instability and a failure to identify and stabilize the patient in a timely manner. This scenario is more common on the general wards, outside of critical care and procedural areas, where patient-to-nurse ratios are higher and monitoring of patients less intense. In this setting, intermittent manual vital sign monitoring with less frequent direct observation by clinicians may increase the likelihood of delayed recognition.

Over the past decade, hospitals in several countries have designed systems to identify and treat early clinical deterioration in patients. The purpose of these rapid response systems is to improve patient outcomes by bringing critical care expertise to patients. The rapid response system has several components:

- Event detection and response triggering arm
- A planned response arm, such as the RRT
- Quality monitoring
- Administrative support

Many rapid response systems allow activation by a nurse, physician, or family member who is concerned that the patient is deteriorating. Some rapid response systems use specific physiologic criteria to determine when to call the team. These parameters may be weighted, combined, and scored as part of an early warning sign system. The following list gives examples of such criteria for adult patients:

- Threatened airway
- Respiratory rate less than 6/min or more than 30/min
- Heart rate less than 40/min or greater than 140/min
- Systolic blood pressure less than 90 mm Hg
- Symptomatic hypertension
- Unexpected decrease in level of consciousness
- Unexplained agitation
- Seizure
- Significant fall in urine output
- Subjective concern about the patient

Medical Emergency Teams and Rapid Response Teams

RRTs, or METs, were established for early intervention in patients whose conditions were deteriorating, with the goal of preventing IHCA.[13,14] They can be composed of varying combinations of physicians, nurses, and respiratory therapists. These teams are usually summoned to patient bedsides when an acute deterioration is recognized by other hospital staff. Monitoring and resuscitation equipment and drug therapies often accompany the team.

The rapid response system is critically dependent on early identification and activation to immediately summon the team to the patient's bedside. These teams typically consist of healthcare providers with both the critical care or emergency care experience and skills to support immediate intervention for life-threatening situations. These teams are responsible for performing a rapid patient assessment and initiating appropriate treatment to reverse physiologic deterioration and prevent a poor outcome.

Published Studies

The majority of published before-and-after studies of METs or rapid response systems have reported a 17% to 65% drop in the rate of cardiac arrests after the intervention. Other documented benefits of these systems include

- A decrease in unplanned emergency transfers to the ICU
- Decreased ICU and total hospital length of stay
- Reductions in postoperative morbidity and mortality rates
- Improved rates of survival from cardiac arrest

The recently published Medical Emergency Response Improvement Team (MERIT) trial is the only randomized controlled trial comparing hospitals with an MET with those without one. The study did not show a difference in the composite primary outcome (cardiac arrest, unexpected death, unplanned ICU admission) between the 12 hospitals in which an MET system was introduced and 11 hospitals that had no MET system in place. Further research is needed about the critical details of implementation and the potential effectiveness of METs in preventing cardiac arrest or improving other important patient outcomes.

Implementation of a Rapid Response System

Implementing any type of rapid response system will require a significant cultural change in most hospitals. Those who design and manage the system must pay particular attention to issues that may prevent the system from being used effectively. Examples of such issues are insufficient resources, poor education, fear of calling the team, fear of losing control over patient care, and resistance from team members.

Implementation of a rapid response system requires ongoing education, impeccable data collection and review, and feedback. Development and maintenance of these programs requires a long-term cultural and financial commitment from the hospital administration. Hospital administrators and healthcare professionals need to reorient their approach to emergency medical events and develop a culture of patient safety with a primary goal of decreasing morbidity and mortality.

Life Is Why

Education Is Why

Heart disease is the No. 1 cause of death in the world—with more than 17 million deaths per year. That's why the AHA is continuously transforming our training solutions as science evolves, and driving awareness of how everyone can help save a life.

References

1. Cummins RO, Ornato JP, Thies WH, Pepe PE. Improving survival from sudden cardiac arrest: the "chain of survival" concept. A statement for health professionals from the Advanced Cardiac Life Support Subcommittee and the Emergency Cardiac Care Committee, American Heart Association. *Circulation.* 1991;83(5):1832-1847.

2. Jacobs I, Nadkarni V, Bahr J, et al; International Liaison Committee on Resuscitation; American Heart Association; European Resuscitation Council; Australian Resuscitation Council; New Zealand Resuscitation Council; Heart and Stroke Foundation of Canada; InterAmerican Heart Foundation; Resuscitation Councils of Southern Africa; ILCOR Task Force on Cardiac Arrest and Cardiopulmonary Resuscitation Outcomes. Cardiac arrest and cardiopulmonary resuscitation outcome reports: update and simplification of the Utstein templates for resuscitation registries: a statement for healthcare professionals from a task force of the International Liaison Committee on Resuscitation (American Heart Association, European Resuscitation Council, Australian Resuscitation Council, New Zealand Resuscitation Council, Heart and Stroke Foundation of Canada, InterAmerican Heart Foundation, Resuscitation Councils of Southern Africa). *Circulation.* 2004;110(21):3385-3397.

3. Cummins RO, Chamberlain D, Hazinski MF, et al. Recommended guidelines for reviewing, reporting, and conducting research on in-hospital resuscitation: the in-hospital "Utstein style." American Heart Association. *Circulation.* 1997;95(8):2213-2239.

4. Meaney PA, Bobrow BJ, Mancini ME, et al; CPR Quality Summit Investigators, the American Heart Association Emergency Cardiovascular Care Committee, the Council on Cardiopulmonary, Critical Care Perioperative Resuscitation. Cardiopulmonary resuscitation quality: [corrected] improving cardiac resuscitation outcomes both inside and outside the hospital: a consensus statement from the American Heart Association. *Circulation.* 2013;128(4):417-435.

5. The National Institute of Neurological Disorders and Stroke rt-PA Stroke Study Group. Tissue plasminogen activator for acute ischemic stroke. *N Engl J Med.* 1995;333(24):1581-1587.

6. Acker JE III, Pancioli AM, Crocco TJ, et al; American Heart Association, American Stroke Association Expert Panel on Emergency Medical Services Systems, Stroke Council. Implementation strategies for emergency medical services within stroke systems of care: a policy statement from the American Heart Association/American Stroke Association Expert Panel on Emergency Medical Services Systems and the Stroke Council. *Stroke.* 2007;38(11):3097-3115.

7. Neumar RW, Nolan JP, Adrie C, et al. Post-cardiac arrest syndrome: epidemiology, pathophysiology, treatment, and prognostication. A consensus statement from the International Liaison Committee on Resuscitation (American Heart Association, Australian and New Zealand Council on Resuscitation, European Resuscitation Council, Heart and Stroke Foundation of Canada, InterAmerican Heart Foundation, Resuscitation Council of Asia, and the Resuscitation Council of Southern Africa); the American Heart Association Emergency Cardiovascular Care Committee; the Council on Cardiovascular Surgery and Anesthesia; the Council on Cardiopulmonary, Perioperative, and Critical Care; the Council on Clinical Cardiology; and the Stroke Council. *Circulation.* 2008;118(23):2452-2483.

8. Carr BG, Kahn JM, Merchant RM, Kramer AA, Neumar RW. Inter-hospital variability in post-cardiac arrest mortality. *Resuscitation.* 2009;80(1):30-34.

9. Callaway CW, Schmicker R, Kampmeyer M, et al. Receiving hospital characteristics associated with survival after out-of-hospital cardiac arrest. *Resuscitation.* 2010;81(5):524-529.

10. Go AS, Mozaffarian D, Roger VL, et al; American Heart Association Statistics Committee, Stroke Statistics Subcommittee. Heart disease and stroke statistics—2013 update: a report from the American Heart Association. *Circulation.* 2013;127(1):e6-e245.

11. Gurses AP, Seidl KL, Vaidya V, et al. Systems ambiguity and guideline compliance: a qualitative study of how intensive care units follow evidence-based guidelines to reduce health-care-associated infections. *Qual Saf Health Care.* 2008;17(5):351-359.

12. Pronovost PJ, Bo-Linn GW. Preventing patient harms through systems of care. *JAMA.* 2012;308(8):769-770.

13. Devita MA, Bellomo R, Hillman K, et al. Findings of the first consensus conference on medical emergency teams. *Crit Care Med.* 2006;34(9):2463-2478.

14. Peberdy MA, Cretikos M, Abella BS, et al; International Liaison Committee on Resuscitation, American Heart Association, Australian Resuscitation Council, European Resuscitation Council, Heart Stroke Foundation of Canada, InterAmerican Heart Foundation, Resuscitation Council of Southern Africa, New Zealand Resuscitation Council, American Heart Association Emergency Cardiovascular Care Committee, American Heart Association Council on Cardiopulmonary Perioperative Critical Care, Interdisciplinary Working Group on Quality of Care and Outcomes Research. Recommended guidelines for monitoring, reporting, and conducting research on medical emergency team, outreach, and rapid response systems: an Utstein-style scientific statement: a scientific statement from the International Liaison Committee on Resuscitation (American Heart Association, Australian Resuscitation Council, European Resuscitation Council, Heart and Stroke Foundation of Canada, InterAmerican Heart Foundation, Resuscitation Council of Southern Africa, and the New Zealand Resuscitation Council); the American Heart Association Emergency Cardiovascular Care Committee; the Council on Cardiopulmonary, Perioperative, and Critical Care; and the Interdisciplinary Working Group on Quality of Care and Outcomes Research. *Circulation.* 2007;116(21):2481-2500.

Effective High-Performance Team Dynamics

Introduction

Successful resuscitation attempts often require healthcare providers to simultaneously perform a variety of interventions. Although a CPR-trained bystander working alone can resuscitate a patient within the first moments after collapse, most attempts require the concerted efforts of multiple healthcare providers. Effective teamwork divides the tasks while multiplying the chances of a successful outcome.

Successful high-performance teams not only have medical expertise and mastery of resuscitation skills, but they also demonstrate effective communication and team dynamics. Part 3 of this manual discusses the importance of team roles, behaviors of effective team leaders and team members, and elements of effective high-performance team dynamics.

During the course, you will have an opportunity to practice performing different roles as a member and as a leader of a simulated high-performance team.

Foundational Facts

Understanding Team Roles

Whether you are a team member or a team leader during a resuscitation attempt, you should **understand not only your role but also the roles of other members.** This awareness will help you anticipate

- What actions will be performed next
- How to communicate and work as a member or as a leader of a high-performance team

---

Roles of the Leader and Members of a High-Performance Team

Role of the Team Leader

The role of the team leader is multifaceted. The team leader

- Organizes the group
- Monitors individual performance of team members
- Backs up team members
- Models excellent team behavior
- Trains and coaches
- Facilitates understanding
- Focuses on comprehensive patient care

Every high-performance team needs a leader to organize the efforts of the group. The team leader is responsible for making sure everything is done at the right time in the right way by monitoring and integrating individual performance of team members. The role of the team leader is similar to that of an orchestra conductor directing individual musicians. Like a conductor, the team leader does not play the instruments but instead knows how each member of the orchestra fits into the overall music.

The role of the team leader also includes modeling excellent team behavior and leadership skills for the team and other people involved or interested in the resuscitation. The team leader should serve as a teacher or guide to help train future team leaders and improve team effectiveness. After resuscitation, the team leader can facilitate analysis, critique, and practice in preparation for the next resuscitation attempt.

The team leader also helps team members understand why they must perform certain tasks in a specific way. The team leader should be able to explain why it is essential to

- Push hard and fast in the center of the chest
- Ensure complete chest recoil
- Minimize interruptions in chest compressions
- Avoid excessive ventilation

Whereas members of a high-performance team should focus on their individual tasks, the team leader must focus on comprehensive patient care.

Role of the Team Member

Team members must be proficient in performing the skills authorized by their scope of practice. It is essential to the success of the resuscitation attempt that members of a high-performance team are

- Clear about role assignments
- Prepared to fulfill their role responsibilities
- Well practiced in resuscitation skills
- Knowledgeable about the algorithms
- Committed to success

Elements of Effective High-Performance Team Dynamics

Roles

Clear Roles and Responsibilities

Every member of the team should know his or her role and responsibilities. Just as different-shaped pieces make up a jigsaw puzzle, each team member's role is unique and critical to the effective performance of the team. Figure 5A identifies 6 team roles for resuscitation. When fewer than 6 people are present, these tasks must be prioritized and assigned to the healthcare providers present. Figure 5B shows how multiple providers can take on high-priority tasks seamlessly as more team members get to the patient.

Positions for 6-Person High-Performance Teams*

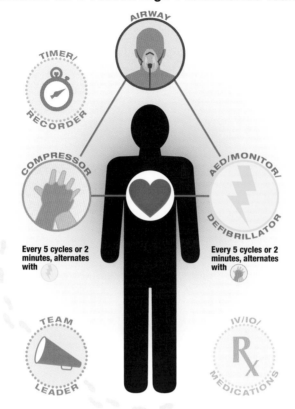

Resuscitation Triangle Roles

Compressor

- Assesses the patient
- Does 5 cycles of chest compressions
- Alternates with AED/Monitor/ Defibrillator every 5 cycles or 2 minutes (or earlier if signs of fatigue set in)

AED/Monitor/ Defibrillator

- Brings and operates the AED/monitor/defibrillator
- Alternates with Compressor every 5 cycles or 2 minutes (or earlier if signs of fatigue set in), ideally during rhythm analysis
- If a monitor is present, places it in a position where it can be seen by the Team Leader (and most of the team)

Airway

- Opens the airway
- Provides bag-mask ventilation
- Inserts airway adjuncts as appropriate

The team owns the code. No team member leaves the triangle except to protect his or her safety.

Every 5 cycles or 2 minutes, alternates with

Every 5 cycles or 2 minutes, alternates with

Leadership Roles

Team Leader

- **Every resuscitation team must have a defined leader**
- Assigns roles to team members
- Makes treatment decisions
- Provides feedback to the rest of the team as needed
- Assumes responsibility for roles not assigned

IV/IO/Medications

- An ACLS provider role
- Initiates IV/IO access
- Administers medications

Timer/Recorder

- Records the time of interventions and medications (and announces when these are next due)
- Records the frequency and duration of interruptions in compressions
- Communicates these to the Team Leader (and the rest of the team)

*This is a suggested team formation. Roles may be adapted to local protocol.

A

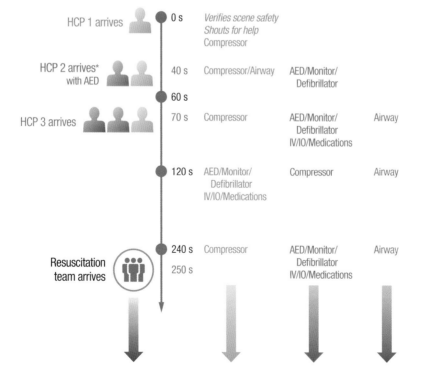

B

Figure 5. A, Suggested locations of team leader and team members during case simulations and clinical events. **B,** Priority-based multiple-rescuer response. This figure illustrates a potential seamless, time-sensitive, integrated team-based approach to resuscitation where roles and interventions are prioritized and distributed as more resources arrive to the patient. Times (in seconds) may vary based on circumstances, response times, and local protocols. *With 2 or more rescuers, one healthcare provider (HCP) should assume the role of team leader.

When roles are unclear, team performance suffers. Signs of unclear roles include

- Performing the same task more than once
- Missing essential tasks
- Team members having multiple roles even if there are enough providers

To avoid inefficiencies, the team leader must clearly delegate tasks. Team members should communicate when and if they can handle additional responsibilities. The team leader should encourage team members to participate in leadership and not simply follow directions blindly.

Do	
Team leader	• Clearly define all team member roles in the clinical setting
Team members	• Seek out and perform clearly defined tasks appropriate to your level of competence • Ask for a new task or role if you are unable to perform your assigned task because it is beyond your level of experience or competence

Don't	
Team leader	• Neglect to assign tasks to all available team members • Assign tasks to team members who are unsure of their responsibilities • Distribute assignments unevenly, leaving some with too much to do and others with too little
Team members	• Avoid taking assignments • Take assignments beyond your level of competence or expertise

Knowing Your Limitations

Not only should everyone on the team know his or her own limitations and capabilities, but the team leader should also be aware of them. This allows the team leader to evaluate team resources and call for backup of team members when assistance is needed. High-performance team members should anticipate situations in which they might require assistance and inform the team leader.

During the stress of an attempted resuscitation, do not practice or explore a new skill. If you need extra help, request it early. It is not a sign of weakness or incompetence to ask for help; it is better to have more help than needed rather than not enough help, which might negatively affect patient outcome.

Do	
Team leader and team members	• Call for assistance early rather than waiting until the patient deteriorates to the point that help is critical • Seek advice from more experienced personnel when the patient's condition worsens despite primary treatment

Don't	
Team leader and team members	• Reject offers from others to carry out an assigned task you are unable to complete, especially if task completion is essential to treatment
Team members	• Use or start an unfamiliar treatment or therapy without seeking advice from more experienced personnel • Take on too many assignments at a time when assistance is readily available

Constructive Interventions

During a resuscitation attempt, the leader or a member of a high-performance team may need to intervene if an action that is about to occur may be inappropriate at the time. Although constructive intervention is necessary, it should be tactful. Team leaders should avoid confrontation with team members. Instead, conduct a debriefing afterward if constructive criticism is needed.

Do	
Team leader	• Ask that a different intervention be started if it has a higher priority
Team members	• Suggest an alternative drug or dose in a confident manner • Question a colleague who is about to make a mistake

Don't	
Team leader	• Fail to reassign a team member who is trying to function beyond his or her level of skill
Team members	• Ignore a team member who is about to administer a drug incorrectly

What to Communicate

Knowledge Sharing

Sharing information is a critical component of effective team performance. Team leaders may become trapped in a specific treatment or diagnostic approach; this common human error is called a *fixation error*. Examples of 3 common types of fixation errors are

"Everything is OK."
"This and only this is the correct path."
"Do anything but this."

When resuscitative efforts are ineffective, go back to the basics and talk as a team, with conversations like, "Well, we've observed the following on the Primary Assessment… Have we missed something?"

Members of a high-performance team should inform the team leader of any changes in the patient's condition to ensure that decisions are made with all available information.

Do	
Team leader	• Encourage an environment of information sharing and ask for suggestions if uncertain of the next best interventions • Ask for good ideas for differential diagnoses • Ask if anything has been overlooked (eg, intravenous access should have been obtained or drugs should have been administered)
Team members	• Share information with other team members

Don't	
Team leader	• Ignore others' suggestions for treatment • Overlook or fail to examine clinical signs that are relevant to the treatment
Team members	• Ignore important information to improve your role

Summarizing and Reevaluating

An essential role of the team leader is monitoring and reevaluating

- The patient's status
- Interventions that have been performed
- Assessment findings

A good practice is for the team leader to summarize this information out loud in a periodic update to the team. Review the status of the resuscitation attempt and announce the plan for the next few steps. Remember that the patient's condition can change. Remain flexible to changing treatment plans and revisiting the initial differential diagnosis. Ask for information and summaries from the timer/recorder as well.

Do	
Team leader	• Draw continuous attention to decisions about differential diagnoses • Review or maintain an ongoing record of drugs and treatments administered and the patient's response
Team leader and team members	• Clearly draw attention to significant changes in the patient's clinical condition • Increase monitoring (eg, frequency of respirations and blood pressure) when the patient's condition deteriorates

Don't	
Team leader	• Fail to change a treatment strategy when new information supports such a change • Fail to inform arriving personnel of the current status and plans for further action

How to Communicate

Closed-Loop Communications

When communicating with high-performance team members, the team leader should use closed-loop communication by taking these steps:

1. The team leader gives a message, order, or assignment to a team member.

2. By receiving a clear response and eye contact, the team leader confirms that the team member heard and understood the message.

3. The team leader listens for confirmation of task performance from the team member before assigning another task.

Do	
Team leader	• Assign another task after receiving oral confirmation that a task has been completed, such as, "Now that the IV is in, give 1 mg of epinephrine"
Team members	• Close the loop: Inform the team leader when a task begins or ends, such as, "The IV is in"

Don't	
Team leader	• Give more tasks to a team member without asking or receiving confirmation of a completed assignment
Team members	• Give drugs without verbally confirming the order with the team leader • Forget to inform the team leader after giving the drug or performing the procedure

Clear Messages

Clear messages consist of concise communication spoken with distinctive speech in a controlled tone of voice. All healthcare providers should deliver messages and orders in a calm and direct manner without yelling or shouting. Unclear communication can lead to unnecessary delays in treatment or to medication errors.

Yelling or shouting can impair effective high-performance team interaction. Only one person should talk at any time.

Do	
Team leader	• Encourage team members to speak clearly
Team members	• Repeat the medication order • Question an order if the slightest doubt exists

Don't	
Team leader	• Mumble or speak in incomplete sentences • Give unclear messages and drug/medication orders • Yell, scream, or shout
Team members	• Feel patronized by distinct and concise messages

Mutual Respect

The best high-performance teams are composed of members who share a mutual respect for each other and work together in a collegial, supportive manner. To have a high-performance team, everyone must abandon ego and respect each other during the resuscitation attempt, regardless of any additional training or experience that the team leader or specific team members may have.

Do

Team leader and team members	• Speak in a friendly, controlled tone of voice • Avoid shouting or displaying aggression if you are not understood initially
Team leader	• Acknowledge correctly completed assignments by saying, "Thanks—good job!"

Don't

Team leader and team members	• Shout or yell at team members—when one person raises his voice, others will respond similarly • Behave aggressively or confuse directive behavior with aggression • Be uninterested in others

Part 4

The Systematic Approach

Introduction

Healthcare providers use a systematic approach to assess and treat arrest and acutely ill or injured patients for optimal care. The goal of the high-performance team's interventions for a patient in respiratory or cardiac arrest is to support and restore effective oxygenation, ventilation, and circulation with return of intact neurologic function. An intermediate goal of resuscitation is return of spontaneous circulation (ROSC). The actions used are guided by the following systematic approaches:

- BLS Assessment
- Primary Assessment (A, B, C, D, and E)
- Secondary Assessment (SAMPLE, H's and T's)

The Systematic Approach

Overview of the Systematic Approach

After determination of scene safety, the systematic approach (Figure 6) first requires ACLS providers to determine the patient's level of consciousness. As you approach the patient,

- If the patient appears unconscious
  - Use the BLS Assessment for the initial evaluation
  - After completing all of the appropriate steps of the BLS Assessment, use the Primary and Secondary Assessments for more advanced evaluation and treatment
- If the patient appears conscious
  - Use the Primary Assessment for your initial evaluation

Before conducting these assessments, make sure the scene is safe.

The Systematic Approach

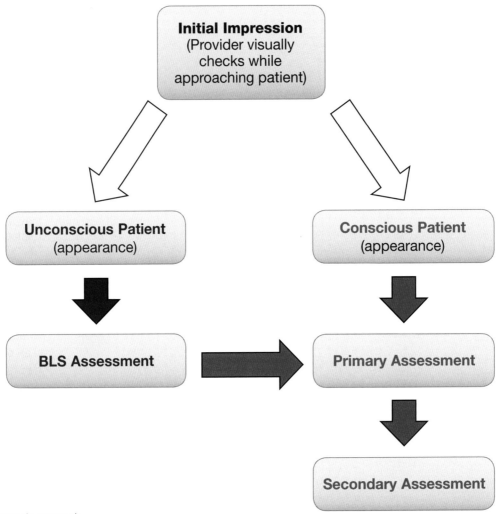

Figure 6. The systematic approach.

The details of the BLS Assessment and Primary and Secondary Assessments are described below.

The BLS Assessment

Foundational Facts

Starting CPR When You Are Not Sure About a Pulse

If you are unsure about the presence of a pulse, begin cycles of compressions and ventilations. Unnecessary compressions are less harmful than failing to provide compressions when needed. Delaying or failing to start CPR in a patient without a pulse reduces the chance of survival.

Overview of the BLS Assessment

The BLS Assessment is a systematic approach to BLS that any trained healthcare provider can perform. This approach stresses *early CPR* and *early defibrillation*. It does not include advanced interventions, such as advanced airway techniques or drug administration. By using the BLS Assessment, healthcare providers may achieve their goal of supporting or restoring effective oxygenation, ventilation, and circulation until ROSC or initiation of ACLS interventions. Performing the actions in the BLS Assessment substantially improves the patient's chance of survival and a good neurologic outcome.

Remember: Assess…then perform appropriate action.

Caution

Agonal Gasps

- Agonal gasps are *not* normal breathing. Agonal gasps may be present in the first minutes after sudden cardiac arrest.
- A patient who gasps usually looks like he is drawing air in very quickly. The mouth may be open and the jaw, head, or neck may move with gasps. Gasps may appear forceful or weak. Some time may pass between gasps because they usually happen at a slow rate. The gasp may sound like a snort, snore, or groan. Gasping is not normal breathing. It is a **sign of cardiac arrest**.

Although the BLS Assessment requires no advanced equipment, healthcare providers can use any readily available universal precaution supplies or adjuncts, such as a bag-mask ventilation device. Whenever possible, place the patient on a firm surface in a supine position to maximize the effectiveness of chest compressions. Table 2 is an overview of the BLS Assessment, and Figures 7 through 11 illustrate the steps needed during the BLS Assessment. Before approaching the patient, ensure scene safety. A rapid scene survey should be performed to determine if any reason exists not to initiate CPR, such as a threat to safety of the provider.

 For more details, watch the High-Quality BLS video on the Student Website (**www.heart.org/eccstudent**).

Table 2. The BLS Assessment

Assess	Assessment Technique and Action	
Check responsiveness	• Tap and shout, *"Are you OK?"*	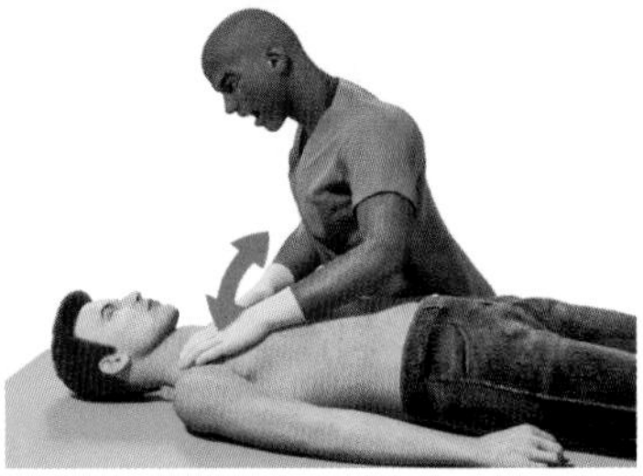 **Figure 7.** Check responsiveness.
Shout for nearby help/ activate the emergency response system and get the AED/defibrillator	• Shout for nearby help • Activate the emergency response system • Get an AED if one is available, or send someone to activate the emergency response system and get an AED or defibrillator	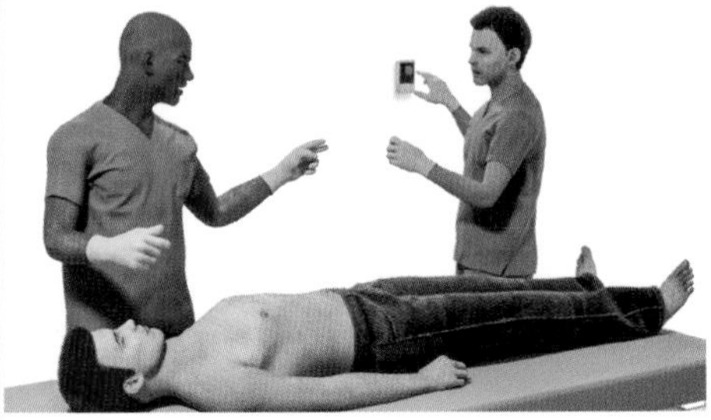 **Figure 8.** Shout for nearby help/activate the emergency response system/get an AED.
Check breathing and pulse	• **Check for absent or abnormal breathing** (no breathing or only gasping) by looking at or **scanning the chest for movement** for about 5 to 10 seconds ***Ideally, the pulse check is performed simultaneously with the breathing check to minimize delay in detection of cardiac arrest and initiation of CPR*** • **Check pulse** for 5 to 10 seconds • If no pulse within 10 seconds, start CPR, beginning with chest compressions • If there is a pulse, start rescue breathing at 1 breath every 5 to 6 seconds. Check pulse about every 2 minutes	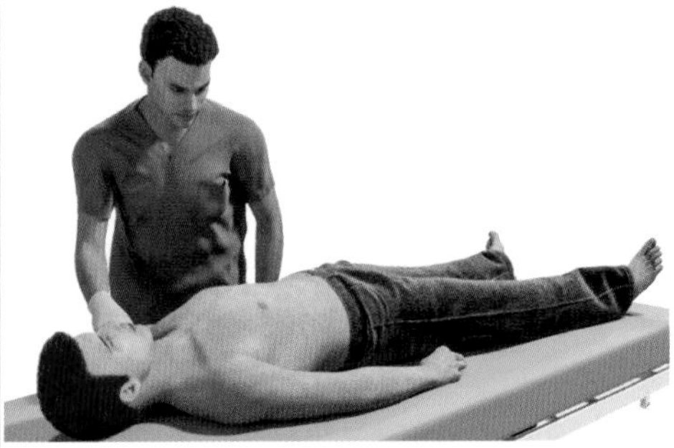 **Figure 9.** Check breathing and pulse simultaneously. 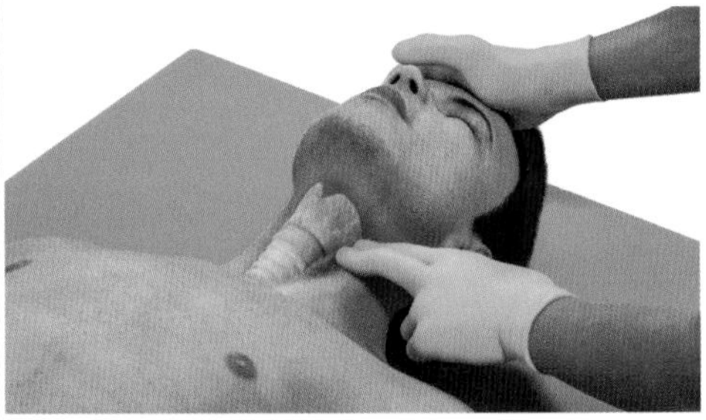 **Figure 10.** Checking a carotid pulse.
Defibrillation	• If no pulse, check for a shockable rhythm with an AED/defibrillator as soon as it arrives • Provide shocks as indicated • Follow each shock immediately with CPR, beginning with compressions	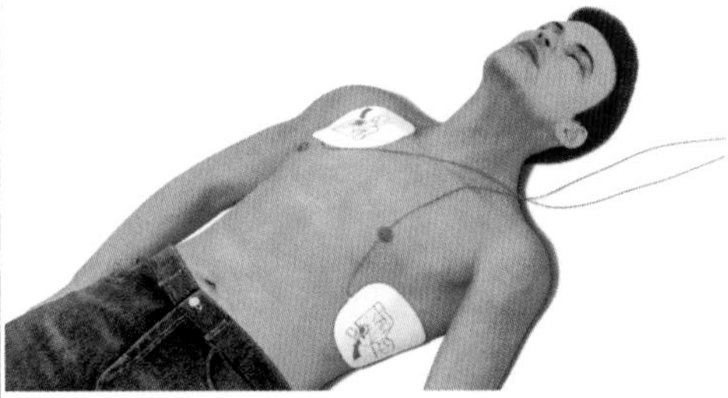 **Figure 11.** Defibrillation.

Minimizing Interruptions

ACLS providers must make every effort to minimize any interruptions in chest compressions. Try to limit interruptions in chest compressions (eg, defibrillation and rhythm analysis) to no longer than 10 seconds, except in extreme circumstances, such as removing the patient from a dangerous environment. When you stop chest compressions, blood flow to the brain and heart stops. See Figure 12.

Avoid:

- Prolonged rhythm analysis
- Frequent or inappropriate pulse checks
- Taking too long to give breaths to the patient
- Unnecessarily moving the patient

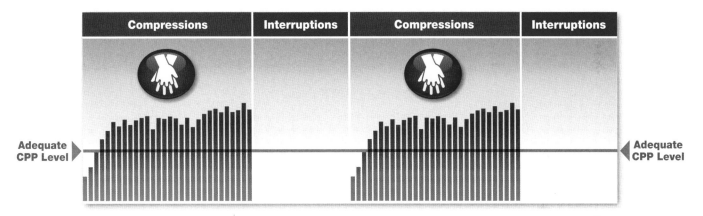

Figure 12. Relationship of quality CPR to coronary perfusion pressure demonstrating the need to minimize interruptions in compressions.

Coronary perfusion pressure (CPP) is aortic relaxation ("diastolic") pressure minus right atrial relaxation ("diastolic") pressure. During CPR, CPP correlates with both myocardial blood flow and ROSC. In 1 human study, ROSC did not occur unless a CPP of 15 mm Hg or greater was achieved during CPR.

Critical Concepts

Quality Compressions

- Compress the chest at least 2 inches (5 cm).
- Compress the chest at a rate of 100 to 120/min.
- Allow complete chest recoil after each compression.

Foundational Facts

Chest Compression Depth

Chest compressions are more often too shallow than too deep. However, research suggests that compression depth greater than 2.4 inches (6 cm) in adults may not be optimal for survival from cardiac arrest and may cause injuries. If you have a CPR quality feedback device, it is optimal to target your compression depth from 2 to 2.4 inches (5 to 6 cm).

Foundational Facts

Single Healthcare Provider May Tailor Response

- Single healthcare providers may tailor the sequence of rescue actions to the most likely cause of arrest. For example, if a lone healthcare provider sees an adolescent suddenly collapse, it is reasonable to assume that the patient has suffered a sudden cardiac arrest.
- A single rescuer should call for help (activate the emergency response system), get an AED (if nearby), return to the patient to attach the AED, and then provide CPR.
- On the other hand, if hypoxia is the presumed cause of the cardiac arrest (such as in a drowning patient), the healthcare provider may give approximately 2 minutes of CPR before activating the emergency response system.

Critical Concepts

High-Quality CPR

- Compress the chest hard and fast.
- Allow complete chest recoil after each compression.
- Minimize interruptions in compressions (10 seconds or less).
- Avoid excessive ventilation.
- Switch compressor about every 2 minutes or earlier if fatigued.*

*Switch should take 5 seconds or less.

The Primary Assessment

Overview of the Primary Assessment

For unconscious patients in arrest (cardiac or respiratory):

- Healthcare providers should conduct the Primary Assessment after completing the BLS Assessment.

For conscious patients who may need more advanced assessment and management techniques:

- Healthcare providers should conduct the Primary Assessment first.

In the Primary Assessment, you continue to assess and perform an action as appropriate until transfer to the next level of care. Many times, members of a high-performance team perform assessments and actions in ACLS simultaneously.

Remember: Assess...then perform appropriate action.

Table 3 provides an overview of the Primary Assessment.

Table 3. The Primary Assessment

Assess	Action as Appropriate

Airway
 	
• *Is the airway patent?*
• *Is an advanced airway indicated?*
• *Is proper placement of airway device confirmed?*
• *Is tube secured and placement reconfirmed frequently?*
	• **Maintain airway patency in unconscious patients** by use of the head tilt–chin lift, oropharyngeal airway, or nasopharyngeal airway
	• **Use advanced airway management if needed** (eg, laryngeal mask airway, laryngeal tube, esophageal-tracheal tube, endotracheal tube)
	
	Healthcare providers must weigh the benefit of advanced airway placement against the adverse effects of interrupting chest compressions. If bag-mask ventilation is adequate, healthcare providers may defer insertion of an advanced airway until the patient does not respond to initial CPR and defibrillation or until spontaneous circulation returns. Advanced airway devices such as a laryngeal mask airway, laryngeal tube, or esophageal-tracheal tube can be placed while chest compressions continue.
	
	If using advanced airway devices:
	• **Confirm proper integration of CPR and ventilation**
	• **Confirm proper placement of advanced airway devices** by
	   – Physical examination
	   – Quantitative waveform capnography
	• **Secure the device to prevent dislodgment**
	• **Monitor airway placement with continuous quantitative waveform capnography**

Breathing
 	
• *Are ventilation and oxygenation adequate?*
• *Are quantitative waveform capnography and oxyhemoglobin saturation monitored?*
	• **Give supplementary oxygen when indicated**
	   – For cardiac arrest patients, administer 100% oxygen
	   – For others, titrate oxygen administration to achieve oxygen saturation values of 94% or greater by pulse oximetry
	• **Monitor the adequacy of ventilation and oxygenation** by
	   – Clinical criteria (chest rise and cyanosis)
	   – Quantitative waveform capnography
	   – Oxygen saturation
	• **Avoid excessive ventilation**

Circulation
 	
• *Are chest compressions effective?*
• *What is the cardiac rhythm?*
• *Is defibrillation or cardioversion indicated?*
• *Has IV/IO access been established?*
• *Is ROSC present?*
• *Is the patient with a pulse unstable?*
• *Are medications needed for rhythm or blood pressure?*
• *Does the patient need volume (fluid) for resuscitation?*
	• **Monitor CPR quality**
	   – Quantitative waveform capnography (if P_{ETCO_2} is less than 10 mm Hg, attempt to improve CPR quality)
	   – Intra-arterial pressure (if relaxation phase [diastolic] pressure is less than 20 mm Hg, attempt to improve CPR quality)
	• **Attach monitor/defibrillator for arrhythmias or cardiac arrest rhythms** (eg, ventricular fibrillation [VF], pulseless ventricular tachycardia [PVT], asystole, pulseless electrical activity [PEA])
	• **Provide defibrillation/cardioversion**
	• **Obtain IV/IO access**
	• **Give appropriate drugs** to manage rhythm and blood pressure
	• **Give IV/IO fluids if needed**
	• **Check glucose and temperature**
	• **Check perfusion issues**

Disability	• **Check for neurologic function** • **Quickly assess for responsiveness, levels of consciousness, and pupil dilation** • **AVPU: Alert, Voice, Painful, Unresponsive**
Exposure	• **Remove clothing to perform a physical examination, looking for obvious signs of trauma, bleeding, burns, unusual markings, or medical alert bracelets**

P_{ETCO_2} is the partial pressure of CO_2 in exhaled air at the end of the exhalation phase.

The Secondary Assessment

Overview of the Secondary Assessment

The Secondary Assessment involves the differential diagnosis, including a focused medical history and searching for and treating underlying causes (H's and T's). Gathering a focused history of the patient is recommended. Ask specific questions related to the patient's presentation. Consider using the memory aid SAMPLE:

Signs and symptoms
Allergies
Medications (including the last dose taken)
Past medical history (especially relating to the current illness)
Last meal consumed
Events

The answers to these questions can help you quickly rule in or rule out suspected diagnoses. Look for and treat the underlying cause by considering the H's and T's to ensure you are not overlooking a dangerous or likely possibility. The H's and T's create a road map for possible diagnoses and interventions for your patient.

H's and T's

Table 4 shows the potential reversible causes of cardiac arrest as well as emergency cardiopulmonary conditions (H's and T's). The ACLS cases provide details on these components.

PEA is associated with many conditions. Healthcare providers should memorize the list of common causes to keep from overlooking an obvious cause of PEA that might be reversed by appropriate treatment.

The most common causes of cardiac arrest are presented as H's and T's in the table below.

Table 4. The Most Common Causes of Cardiac Arrest

H's	T's
Hypovolemia	Tension pneumothorax
Hypoxia	Tamponade (cardiac)
Hydrogen ion (acidosis)	Toxins
Hypo-/hyperkalemia	Thrombosis (pulmonary)
Hypothermia	Thrombosis (coronary)

Critical Concepts

Common Underlying Causes of PEA

- Hypovolemia and hypoxia are the 2 most common underlying and potentially reversible causes of PEA.
- Be sure to look for evidence of these problems as you assess the patient.

Diagnosing and Treating Underlying Causes

Introduction

Patients in cardiac arrest (VF/pVT/asystole/PEA) need rapid assessment and management. Cardiac arrest may be caused by an underlying and potentially reversible problem. If you can quickly identify a specific condition that has caused or is contributing to PEA and correct it, you may achieve ROSC. The identification of the underlying cause is of paramount importance in cases of PEA and asystole.

In the search for the underlying cause, do the following:

- Consider frequent causes of PEA by recalling the H's and T's
- Analyze the ECG for clues to the underlying cause
- Recognize hypovolemia
- Recognize drug overdose/poisonings

Conditions and Management

The **H's and T's** are a memory aid for the most common and potentially reversible causes of periarrest and cardiopulmonary arrest (Table 4).

Hypovolemia

Hypovolemia, a common cause of PEA, initially produces the classic physiologic response of a *rapid, narrow-complex tachycardia (sinus tachycardia)* and typically produces increased diastolic and decreased systolic pressures. As loss of blood volume continues, blood pressure drops, eventually becoming undetectable, but the narrow QRS complexes and rapid rate continue (ie, PEA).

You should consider hypovolemia as a cause of hypotension, which can deteriorate to PEA. Providing prompt treatment can reverse the pulseless state by rapidly correcting the hypovolemia. Common nontraumatic causes of hypovolemia include occult internal hemorrhage and severe dehydration. Consider volume infusion for PEA associated with a narrow-complex tachycardia.

Cardiac and Pulmonary Conditions

Acute coronary syndromes involving a large amount of heart muscle can present as PEA. That is, occlusion of the left main or proximal left anterior descending coronary artery can present with cardiogenic shock rapidly progressing to cardiac arrest and PEA. However, in patients with cardiac arrest and without known pulmonary embolism (PE), routine fibrinolytic treatment given during CPR shows no benefit and is not recommended.

Massive or saddle PE obstructs flow to the pulmonary vasculature and causes acute right heart failure. In patients with cardiac arrest due to presumed or known PE, it is reasonable to administer fibrinolytics.

Pericardial tamponade may be a reversible condition. In the periarrest period, volume infusion in this condition may help while definitive therapy is initiated. Tension pneumothorax can be effectively treated once recognized.

Note that cardiac tamponade, tension pneumothorax, and massive PE cannot be treated unless recognized. Bedside ultrasound, when performed by a skilled provider, may aid in rapid identification of tamponade and PE. There is growing evidence that pneumothorax can be identified by using bedside ultrasound as well. Treatment for cardiac tamponade may require pericardiocentesis. Tension pneumothorax requires needle aspiration and chest tube placement. These procedures are beyond the scope of the ACLS Provider Course.

Drug Overdoses or Toxic Exposures

Certain drug overdoses and toxic exposures may lead to peripheral vascular dilatation and/or myocardial dysfunction with resultant hypotension. The approach to poisoned patients should be aggressive because the toxic effects may progress rapidly and may be of limited duration. In these situations, myocardial dysfunction and arrhythmias may be reversible. Numerous case reports confirm the success of many specific limited interventions with one thing in common: they buy time.

Treatments that can provide this level of support include

- Prolonged basic CPR in special resuscitation situations
- Extracorporeal CPR
- Intra-aortic balloon pumping
- Renal dialysis
- Intravenous lipid emulsion
- Specific drug antidotes (digoxin immune Fab, glucagon, bicarbonate)
- Transcutaneous pacing
- Correction of severe electrolyte disturbances (potassium, magnesium, calcium, acidosis)
- Specific adjunctive agents

Remember, if the patient shows signs of ROSC, post–cardiac arrest care should be initiated.

Part 5

The ACLS Cases

Overview of the Cases

The ACLS simulated cases are designed to review the knowledge and skills you need to successfully participate in course events and pass the Megacode skills test. Each case contains the following topics:

- Introduction
- Rhythms and drugs
- Descriptions or definitions of key concepts
- Overview of algorithm
- Algorithm figure
- Application of the algorithm to the case
- Other related topics

This part contains the following cases:

- Respiratory Arrest
- Acute Coronary Syndromes
  - STEMI
- Acute Stroke
- Cardiac Arrest
  - VF/Pulseless VT
  - Asystole
  - PEA
- Bradycardia
- Tachycardia (Stable and Unstable)
- Immediate Post–Cardiac Arrest Care

Respiratory Arrest Case

Introduction

This case reviews appropriate assessment, intervention, and management options for an *unconscious, unresponsive adult patient in respiratory arrest. Respirations are completely absent or clearly inadequate to maintain effective oxygenation and ventilation. A pulse is present.* (Do not confuse agonal gasps with adequate respirations.) The BLS Assessment and the Primary and Secondary Assessments are used even though the patient is in respiratory arrest and not in cardiac arrest.

Case Drugs

This case involves the following drugs:

- Oxygen

Systems or facilities using rapid sequence intubation may consider additional drugs.

Normal and Abnormal Breathing

The average respiratory rate for an adult is about 12 to 16/min. Normal tidal volume of 8 to 10 mL/kg maintains normal oxygenation and elimination of CO_2.

Tachypnea is a respiratory rate above 20/min and bradypnea is a respiratory rate below 12/min. A respiratory rate below 6/min (hypoventilation) requires assisted ventilation with a bag-mask device or advanced airway with 100% oxygen.

Identification of Respiratory Problems by Severity

Identifying the severity of a respiratory problem will help you decide the most appropriate interventions. Be alert for signs of

- Respiratory distress
- Respiratory failure

Respiratory Distress

Respiratory distress is a clinical state characterized by abnormal respiratory rate (eg, tachypnea) or effort. The respiratory effort may be increased (eg, nasal flaring, retractions, and use of accessory muscles) or inadequate (eg, hypoventilation or bradypnea).

Respiratory distress can range from mild to severe. For example, a patient with mild tachypnea and a mild increase in respiratory effort with changes in airway sounds is in *mild* respiratory distress. A patient with marked tachypnea, significantly increased respiratory effort, deterioration in skin color, and changes in mental status is in *severe* respiratory distress. Severe respiratory distress can be an indication of respiratory failure.

Clinical signs of respiratory distress typically include some or all of the following:

- Tachypnea
- Increased respiratory effort (eg, nasal flaring, retractions)
- Inadequate respiratory effort (eg, hypoventilation or bradypnea)
- Abnormal airway sounds (eg, stridor, wheezing, grunting)
- Tachycardia
- Pale, cool skin (note that some causes of respiratory distress, like sepsis, may cause the skin to get warm, red, and diaphoretic)
- Changes in level of consciousness/agitation
- Use of abdominal muscles to assist in breathing

These indicators may vary in severity.

Respiratory distress is apparent when a patient tries to maintain adequate gas exchange despite airway obstruction, reduced lung compliance, or lung tissue disease. As the patient tires or as respiratory function or effort or both deteriorate, adequate gas exchange cannot be maintained. When this happens, clinical signs of respiratory failure develop.

Respiratory Failure

Respiratory failure is a clinical state of inadequate oxygenation, ventilation, or both. Respiratory failure is often the end stage of respiratory distress. If there is abnormal central nervous system control of breathing or muscle weakness, the patient may show little or no respiratory effort despite being in respiratory failure. In these situations, you may need to identify respiratory failure based on clinical findings. Confirm the diagnosis with objective measurements, such as pulse oximetry or blood gas analysis.

Suspect *probable respiratory failure* if some of the following signs are present:

- Marked tachypnea
- Bradypnea, apnea (late)
- Increased, decreased, or no respiratory effort
- Poor to absent distal air movement
- Tachycardia (early)
- Bradycardia (late)
- Cyanosis
- Stupor, coma (late)

Respiratory failure can result from upper or lower airway obstruction, lung tissue disease, and disordered control of breathing (eg, apnea or shallow, slow respirations). *When respiratory effort is inadequate, respiratory failure can occur without typical signs of respiratory distress.* Respiratory failure is a clinical state that *requires intervention* to prevent deterioration to cardiac arrest. Respiratory failure can occur with a rise in arterial carbon dioxide levels (hypercapnia), a drop in blood oxygenation (hypoxemia), or both.

Respiratory Arrest

Respiratory arrest is the cessation (absence) of breathing. Respiratory arrest is usually caused by an event such as drowning or head injury. For an adult in respiratory arrest, providing a tidal volume of approximately 500 to 600 mL (6 to 7 mL/kg) should suffice. This is consistent with a tidal volume that produces visible chest rise.

Patients with airway obstruction or poor lung compliance may require high pressures to be properly ventilated (to make the chest visibly rise). A pressure-relief valve on a resuscitation bag-mask device may prevent the delivery of a sufficient tidal volume in these patients. Ensure that the bag-mask device allows you to bypass the pressure-relief valve and use high pressures, if necessary, to achieve visible chest expansion.

Excessive ventilation is unnecessary and can cause gastric inflation and its resultant complications, such as regurgitation and aspiration. More important, excessive ventilation can be harmful because it increases intrathoracic pressure, decreases venous return to the heart, and diminishes cardiac output and survival. Healthcare providers should avoid excessive ventilation (too many breaths or too large a volume) during respiratory arrest and cardiac arrest.

The BLS Assessment

When evaluating a patient, proceed with the BLS Assessment after determining that the scene is safe as described in "Part 4: The Systematic Approach."

Assess and Reassess the Patient

The systematic approach is *assessment,* then *action*, for each step in the sequence.

Remember: Assess...then perform appropriate action.

In this case, you assess and find that the patient has a pulse, so you do not use the AED or begin chest compressions.

Ventilation and Pulse Check

In the case of a patient in respiratory arrest with a pulse, deliver ventilations once every 5 to 6 seconds with a bag-mask device or any advanced airway device. Recheck the pulse about every 2 minutes. Take at least 5 seconds but no more than 10 seconds for a pulse check.

The Primary Assessment

Airway Management in Respiratory Arrest

If bag-mask ventilation is adequate, providers may defer insertion of an advanced airway. Healthcare providers should make the decision to place an advanced airway during the Primary Assessment.

Advanced airway equipment includes the laryngeal mask airway, the laryngeal tube, the esophageal-tracheal tube, and the endotracheal (ET) tube. If it is within your scope of practice, you may use advanced airway equipment in the course when appropriate and available.

Ventilations

In this case, the patient is in respiratory arrest but continues to have a pulse. You should ventilate the patient **once every 5 to 6 seconds**. Each breath should take 1 second and achieve visible chest rise. Be careful to avoid excessive ventilation (too many breaths per minute or too large a volume per breath).

FYI 2015 Guidelines

Correct Placement of ET Tube

The AHA recommends continuous waveform capnography in addition to clinical assessment as the most reliable method of confirming and monitoring correct placement of an ET tube.

Management of Respiratory Arrest

Overview

Management of respiratory arrest includes both BLS and ACLS interventions. These interventions may include

- Giving supplementary oxygen
- Opening the airway
- Providing basic ventilation
- Using basic airway adjuncts (OPA and NPA)
- Suctioning

According to the 2015 AHA Guidelines Update for CPR and ECC, *for patients with a perfusing rhythm, ventilations should be delivered once every 5 to 6 seconds.*

Critical Concepts

Avoiding Excessive Ventilation

When using any form of assisted ventilation, you must avoid delivering excessive ventilation (too many breaths per minute or too large a volume per breath). Excessive ventilation can be harmful because it increases intrathoracic pressure, decreases venous return to the heart, and diminishes cardiac output. It may also cause gastric inflation and predispose the patient to vomiting and aspiration of gastric contents. **In addition, hyperventilation may cause cerebral vasoconstriction, reducing blood flow to the brain.**

Giving Supplementary Oxygen

Maintain Oxygen Saturation

Give oxygen to patients with acute cardiac symptoms or respiratory distress. Monitor oxygen saturation and titrate supplementary oxygen to maintain a saturation of 94% or greater. For patients in respiratory or cardiac arrest, striving for 100% oxygen would be more appropriate.

 See the Student Website (**www.heart.org/eccstudent**) for details on use of oxygen in patients not in respiratory or cardiac arrest.

Opening the Airway

Common Cause of Airway Obstruction

Figure 13 demonstrates the anatomy of the airway. The most common cause of upper airway obstruction in the unconscious/unresponsive patient is loss of tone in the throat muscles. In this case, the tongue falls back and occludes the airway at the level of the pharynx (Figure 14A).

Basic Airway Opening Techniques

Basic airway opening techniques will effectively relieve airway obstruction caused either by the tongue or from relaxation of muscles in the upper airway. The basic airway opening technique is head tilt with anterior displacement of the mandible, ie, head tilt–chin lift (Figure 14B).

In the trauma patient with suspected neck injury, use a jaw thrust without head extension (Figure 14C). Because maintaining an open airway and providing ventilation is a priority, use a head tilt–chin lift maneuver if the jaw thrust does not open the airway. ACLS providers should be aware that current BLS training courses teach the jaw-thrust technique to healthcare providers but not to lay rescuers.

Airway Management

Proper airway positioning may be all that is required for patients who can breathe spontaneously. In patients who are unconscious with no cough or gag reflex, insert an OPA or NPA to maintain airway patency.

If you find an unconscious/unresponsive patient who was known to be choking and is now unresponsive and in respiratory arrest, open the mouth wide and look for a foreign object. If you see one, remove it with your fingers. If you do not see a foreign object, begin CPR. Each time you open the airway to give breaths, open the mouth wide and look for a foreign object. Remove it with your fingers if present. If there is no foreign object, resume CPR.

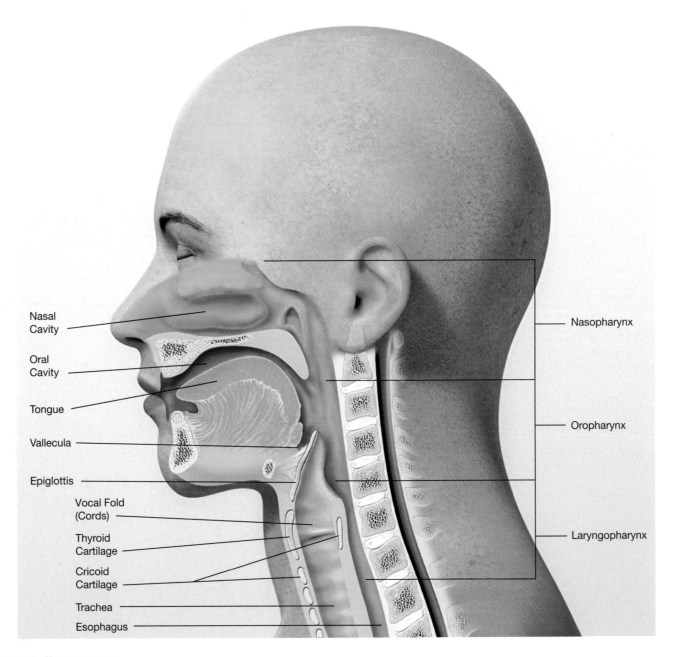

Nasal Cavity

Oral Cavity

Tongue

Vallecula

Epiglottis

Vocal Fold (Cords)

Thyroid Cartilage

Cricoid Cartilage

Trachea

Esophagus

Nasopharynx

Oropharynx

Laryngopharynx

Figure 13. Airway anatomy.

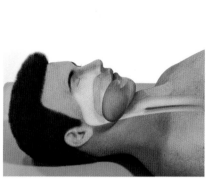
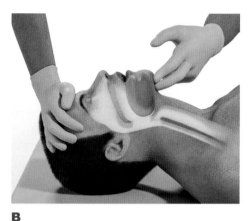
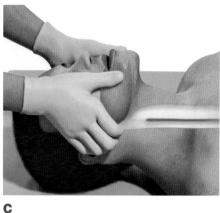

A **B** **C**

Figure 14. Obstruction of the airway by the tongue and epiglottis. When a patient is unresponsive, the tongue can obstruct the airway. The head tilt–chin lift relieves obstruction in the unresponsive patient. **A,** The tongue is obstructing the airway. **B,** The head tilt–chin lift lifts the tongue, relieving the obstruction. **C,** If cervical spine trauma is suspected, healthcare providers should use the jaw thrust without head extension.

Providing Basic Ventilation

Basic Airway Skills

Basic airway skills used to ventilate a patient are

- Head tilt–chin lift
- Jaw thrust without head extension (suspected cervical spine trauma)
- Mouth-to-mouth ventilation
- Mouth-to-nose ventilation
- Mouth-to–barrier device (using a pocket mask) ventilation
- Bag-mask ventilation (Figures 15 and 16)

Bag-Mask Ventilation

A bag-mask ventilation device consists of a ventilation bag attached to a face mask. These devices have been a mainstay of emergency ventilation for decades. Bag-mask devices are the most common method of providing positive-pressure ventilation. When using a bag-mask device, deliver approximately 600 mL tidal volume sufficient to produce chest rise over 1 second. Bag-mask ventilation is not the recommended method of ventilation for a single healthcare provider during CPR. (A single healthcare provider should use a pocket mask to give ventilation, if available.) It is easier for 2 trained and experienced rescuers to provide bag-mask ventilation. One rescuer opens the airway and seals the mask to the face while the other squeezes the bag, with both rescuers watching for visible chest rise.

The universal connections present on all airway devices allow you to connect any ventilation bag to numerous adjuncts. Valves and ports may include

- One-way valves to prevent the patient from rebreathing exhaled air
- Oxygen ports for administering supplementary oxygen
- Medication ports for administering aerosolized and other medications
- Suction ports for clearing the airway
- Ports for quantitative sampling of end-tidal CO_2

You can attach other adjuncts to the patient end of the valve, including a pocket face mask, laryngeal mask airway, laryngeal tube, esophageal-tracheal tube, and ET tube.

 See the Student Website (**www.heart.org/eccstudent**) for more information on bag-mask ventilation.

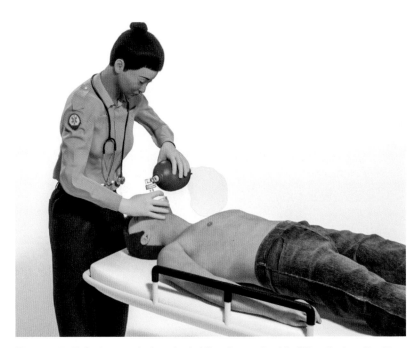

Figure 15. E-C clamp technique for holding the mask while lifting the jaw. Position yourself at the patient's head. Circle the thumb and first finger around the top of the mask (forming a "C") while using the third, fourth, and fifth fingers (forming an "E") to lift the jaw.

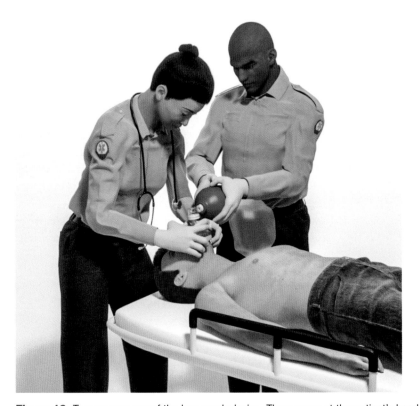

Figure 16. Two-rescuer use of the bag-mask device. The rescuer at the patient's head tilts the patient's head and seals the mask against the patient's face, with the thumb and first finger of each hand creating a "C," to provide a complete seal around the edges of the mask. The rescuer uses the remaining 3 fingers (the "E") to lift the jaw (this holds the airway open). The second rescuer slowly squeezes the bag (over 1 second) until the chest rises. Both providers should observe chest rise.

Basic Airway Adjuncts: Oropharyngeal Airway

Introduction

The OPA is used in patients who are at risk for developing airway obstruction from the tongue or from relaxed upper airway muscles. This J-shaped device (Figure 17A) fits over the tongue to hold it and the soft hypopharyngeal structures away from the posterior wall of the pharynx.

The OPA is used in *unconscious* patients if procedures to open the airway (eg, head tilt–chin lift or jaw thrust) fail to provide and maintain a clear, unobstructed airway. *An OPA should not be used in a conscious or semiconscious patient* because it may stimulate gagging and vomiting. The key assessment is to check whether the patient has an intact cough and gag reflex. If so, do not use an OPA.

The OPA may be used to keep the airway open during bag-mask ventilation when providers might unknowingly push down on the chin, blocking the airway. The OPA is also used during suctioning of the mouth and throat and in intubated patients to prevent them from biting and occluding the ET tube.

Technique of OPA Insertion

Step	Action
1	**Clear the mouth and pharynx** of secretions, blood, or vomit by using a rigid pharyngeal suction tip if possible.
2	**Select the proper size OPA.** Place the OPA against the side of the face (Figure 17B). When the flange of the OPA is at the corner of the mouth, the tip is at the angle of the mandible. A properly sized and inserted OPA results in proper alignment with the glottic opening.
3	**Insert the OPA** so that it curves upward toward the hard palate as it enters the mouth.
4	As the OPA passes through the oral cavity and approaches the posterior wall of the pharynx, **rotate it 180°** into the proper position (Figure 17C). The OPA can also be inserted at a 90° angle to the mouth and then turned down toward the posterior pharynx as it is advanced. In both methods, the goal is to curve the device around the tongue so that the tongue is not inadvertently pushed back into the pharynx rather than being pulled forward by the OPA. An **alternative method** is to insert the OPA straight in while using a tongue depressor or similar device to hold the tongue forward as the OPA is advanced.

After insertion of an OPA, monitor the patient. Keep the head and jaw positioned properly to maintain a patent airway. Suction the airway as needed.

Caution

Be Aware of the Following When Using an OPA

- OPAs that are *too large* may obstruct the larynx or cause trauma to the laryngeal structures.
- OPAs that are *too small* or inserted improperly may push the base of the tongue posteriorly and obstruct the airway.
- Insert the OPA carefully to avoid soft tissue trauma to the lips and tongue.

Remember to use the OPA only in the unresponsive patient with *no cough or gag reflex.* If the patient has a cough or gag reflex, the OPA may stimulate vomiting and laryngospasm.

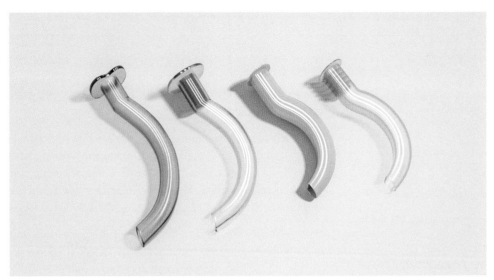

A

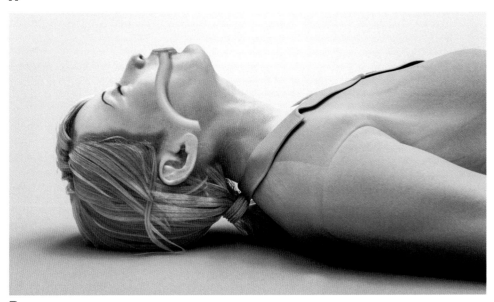

B

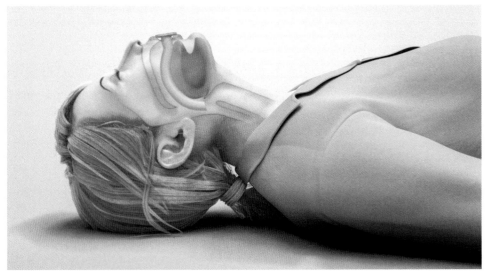

C

Figure 17. Oropharyngeal airways. **A,** Oropharyngeal airway devices. **B,** Oropharyngeal airway device measurement. **C,** Oropharyngeal airway device inserted.

Basic Airway Adjuncts: Nasopharyngeal Airway

Introduction

The NPA is used as an alternative to an OPA in patients who need a basic airway management adjunct. The NPA is a soft rubber or plastic uncuffed tube (Figure 18A) that provides a conduit for airflow between the nares and the pharynx.

Unlike oral airways, NPAs *may be used in conscious, semiconscious, or unconscious patients* (patients with an intact cough and gag reflex). The NPA is indicated when insertion of an OPA is technically difficult or dangerous. Examples include patients with a gag reflex, trismus, massive trauma around the mouth, or wiring of the jaws. The NPA may also be used in patients who are neurologically impaired with poor pharyngeal tone or coordination leading to upper airway obstruction.

Technique of NPA Insertion

Step	Action
1	**Select the proper size NPA.** • Compare the outer circumference of the NPA with the inner aperture of the nares. The NPA should not be so large that it causes sustained blanching of the nostrils. Some providers use the diameter of the patient's smallest finger as a guide to selecting the proper size. • The length of the NPA should be the same as the distance from the tip of the patient's nose to the earlobe (Figure 18B).
2	**Lubricate the airway** with a water-soluble lubricant or anesthetic jelly.
3	**Insert the airway** through the nostril in a posterior direction perpendicular to the plane of the face. Pass it gently along the floor of the nasopharynx (Figure 18C). If you encounter resistance: • Slightly rotate the tube to facilitate insertion at the angle of the nasal passage and nasopharynx. • Attempt placement through the other nostril because patients have different-sized nasal passages.

Reevaluate frequently. Maintain head tilt by providing anterior displacement of the mandible by using a chin lift or jaw thrust. Mucus, blood, vomit, or the soft tissues of the pharynx can obstruct the NPA, which has a small internal diameter. *Frequent evaluation and suctioning of the airway may be necessary to ensure patency.*

Caution

Be Aware of the Following When Using an NPA

• Take care to insert the airway gently to avoid complications. The airway can irritate the mucosa or lacerate adenoidal tissue and cause bleeding, with possible aspiration of clots into the trachea. Suction may be necessary to remove blood or secretions.
• An improperly sized NPA may enter the esophagus. With active ventilation, such as bag-mask ventilation, the NPA may cause gastric inflation and possible hypoventilation.
• An NPA may cause laryngospasm and vomiting, even though it is commonly tolerated by semiconscious patients.
• Use caution in patients with facial trauma because of the risk of misplacement into the cranial cavity through a fractured cribriform plate.

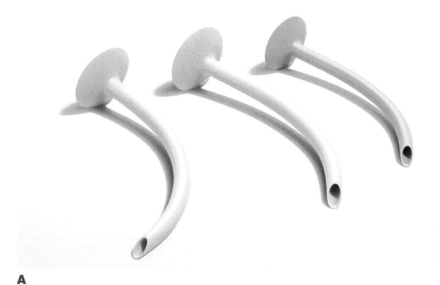

A

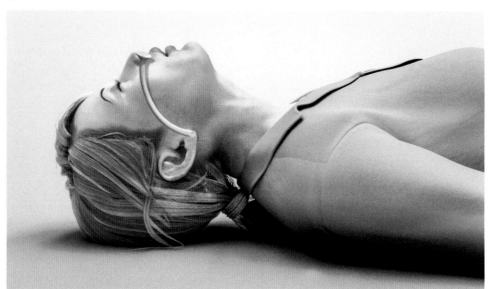

B

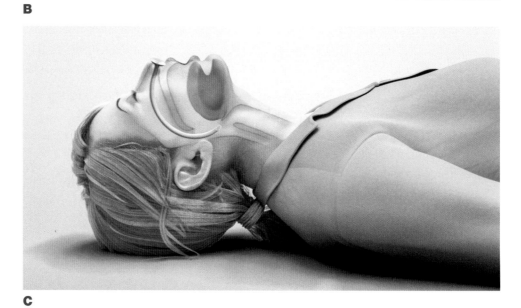

C

Figure 18. Nasopharyngeal airways. **A,** Nasopharyngeal airway devices. **B,** Nasopharyngeal airway device measurement. **C,** Nasopharyngeal airway device inserted.

Caution 	**Precautions for OPAs and NPAs** Take the following precautions when using an OPA or NPA: • Always check spontaneous respirations immediately after insertion of either an OPA or an NPA. • If respirations are absent or inadequate, start positive-pressure ventilations at once with an appropriate device. • If adjuncts are unavailable, use mouth-to-mask barrier device ventilation.

Suctioning

Introduction	Suctioning is an essential component of maintaining a patient's airway. Providers should suction the airway immediately if there are copious secretions, blood, or vomit. Suction devices consist of both portable and wall-mounted units. • Portable suction devices are easy to transport but may not provide adequate suction power. A suction force of −80 to −120 mm Hg is generally necessary. • Wall-mounted suction units should be capable of providing an airflow of greater than 40 L/min at the end of the delivery tube and a vacuum of more than −300 mm Hg when the tube is clamped at full suction. • Adjust the amount of suction force for use in children and intubated patients.
Soft vs Rigid Catheters	Both soft flexible and rigid suctioning catheters are available. *Soft flexible catheters* may be used in the mouth or nose. Soft flexible catheters are available in sterile wrappers and can also be used for ET tube deep suctioning. *Rigid catheters* (eg, Yankauer) are used to suction the oropharynx. These are better for suctioning thick secretions and particulate matter.

Catheter Type	Use for
Soft	• Aspiration of thin secretions from the oropharynx and nasopharynx • Performing intratracheal suctioning • Suctioning through an in-place airway (ie, NPA) to access the back of the pharynx in a patient with clenched teeth
Rigid	• More effective suctioning of the oropharynx, particularly if there is thick particulate matter

Oropharyngeal Suctioning Procedure

Follow the steps below to perform oropharyngeal suctioning.

Step	Action
1	• Measure the catheter before suctioning and do not insert it any further than the distance from the tip of the nose to the earlobe. • Gently insert the suction catheter or device into the oropharynx beyond the tongue.
2	• Apply suction by occluding the side opening of the catheter while withdrawing with a rotating or twisting motion. • If using a rigid suction device (eg, Yankauer suction), place the tip gently into the oral cavity. Advance by pushing the tongue down to reach the oropharynx if necessary.

Endotracheal Tube Suctioning Procedure

Patients with pulmonary secretions may require suctioning even after ET intubation. Follow the steps below to perform ET tube suctioning:

Step	Action
1	• Use sterile technique to reduce the likelihood of airway contamination.
2	• Gently insert the catheter into the ET tube. Be sure the side opening is not occluded during insertion. • Insertion of the catheter beyond the tip of the ET tube is not recommended because it may injure the ET mucosa or stimulate coughing or bronchospasm.
3	• Apply suction by occluding the side opening only while withdrawing the catheter with a rotating or twisting motion. • **Suction attempts should not exceed 10 seconds.** To avoid hypoxemia, precede and follow suctioning attempts with a short period of administration of 100% oxygen.

Monitor the patient's heart rate, pulse, oxygen saturation, and clinical appearance during suctioning. If bradycardia develops, oxygen saturation drops, or clinical appearance deteriorates, interrupt suctioning at once. Administer high-flow oxygen until the heart rate returns to normal and the clinical condition improves. Assist ventilation as needed.

Providing Ventilation With an Advanced Airway

Introduction

Selection of an advanced airway device depends on the training, scope of practice, and equipment of the providers on the high-performance team. Advanced airways include but are not limited to

- Laryngeal mask airway
- Laryngeal tube
- Esophageal-tracheal tube
- ET tube

Because a small proportion of patients cannot be ventilated with a laryngeal mask airway, providers who use this device should have an alternative airway management strategy. A bag-mask device can be this alternate strategy.

This course will familiarize you with types of advanced airways. Instruction in the skilled placement of these airways is beyond the scope of the basic ACLS Provider Course. To be proficient in the use of advanced airway devices, you must have adequate initial training and ongoing experience. Providers who insert advanced airways must participate in a process of CQI to document and minimize complications.

In this course, you will practice ventilating with an advanced airway in place and integrating ventilation with chest compressions.

Ventilation Rates

Airway Devices	Ventilation During Cardiac Arrest	Ventilation During Respiratory Arrest
Any advanced airway	Once every 6 seconds	Once every 5 to 6 seconds

Laryngeal Mask Airway

The laryngeal mask airway is an advanced airway alternative to ET intubation and provides comparable ventilation. It is acceptable to use the laryngeal mask airway as an alternative to an ET tube for airway management in cardiac arrest. *Only experienced providers should perform laryngeal mask airway insertion.*

 See the Student Website (**www.heart.org/eccstudent**) for more information on the laryngeal mask airway.

Laryngeal Tube

The advantages of the laryngeal tube are similar to those of the esophageal-tracheal tube; however, the laryngeal tube is more compact and less complicated to insert.

Healthcare professionals trained in the use of the laryngeal tube may consider it as an alternative to bag-mask ventilation or ET intubation for airway management in cardiac arrest. *Only experienced providers should perform laryngeal tube insertion.*

 See the Laryngeal Intubation section on the Student Website (**www.heart.org/eccstudent**) for more information on this procedure.

Esophageal-Tracheal Tube

The esophageal-tracheal tube is an advanced airway alternative to ET intubation. This device provides adequate ventilation comparable to an ET tube. It is acceptable to use the esophageal-tracheal tube as an alternative to an ET tube for airway management in cardiac arrest.. *Only providers experienced with its use should perform esophageal-tracheal tube insertion.*

 See the Student Website (**www.heart.org/eccstudent**) for more information on the esophageal-tracheal tube.

Endotracheal Tube

A brief summary of the basic steps for performing ET intubation is given here to familiarize the ACLS provider who may assist with the procedure.

- Prepare for intubation by assembling the necessary equipment.
- Perform ET intubation (see the Student Website).
- Inflate cuff or cuffs on the tube.
- Attach the ventilation bag.
- Confirm correct placement by physical examination and a confirmation device. Continuous waveform capnography is recommended (in addition to clinical assessment) as the most reliable method of confirming and monitoring correct placement of an ET tube. Healthcare providers may use colorimetric and nonwaveform carbon dioxide detectors when waveform capnography is not available.
- Secure the tube in place.
- Monitor for displacement.

Only experienced providers should perform ET intubation.

 See the Endotracheal Intubation section on the Student Website (**www.heart.org/eccstudent**) for more information on this procedure.

Caution

Use of Cricoid Pressure

- The routine use of cricoid pressure in cardiac arrest is not recommended.
- Cricoid pressure in nonarrest patients may offer some measure of protection to the airway from aspiration and gastric insufflation during bag-mask ventilation. However, it also may impede ventilation and interfere with placement of a supraglottic airway or intubation.

Precautions for Trauma Patients

Summary

When providing assisted ventilation for patients with known or suspected cervical spine trauma, avoid unnecessary spine movement. Excessive head and neck movement in patients with an unstable cervical spinal column can cause irreversible injury to the spinal cord or worsen a minor spinal cord injury. Approximately 2% of patients with blunt trauma serious enough to require spinal imaging in the ED have a spinal injury. This risk is tripled if the patient has a head or facial injury. Assume that any patient with multiple trauma, head injury, or facial trauma has a spine injury. Be particularly cautious if a patient has suspected cervical spine injury. Examples are patients who have been involved in a high-speed motor vehicle collision, have fallen from a height, or were injured while diving.

Follow these precautions if you suspect cervical spine trauma:

- Open the airway by using a jaw thrust *without head extension*. Because maintaining a patent airway and providing adequate ventilation are priorities, use a head tilt–chin lift maneuver if the jaw thrust is not effective.
- Have another team member stabilize the head in a neutral position during airway manipulation. **Use manual spinal motion restriction rather than immobilization devices.** Manual spinal immobilization is safer. Cervical collars may complicate airway management and may even interfere with airway patency.
- Spinal immobilization devices are helpful during transport.

Acute Coronary Syndromes Case

Introduction

The ACLS provider must have the basic knowledge to assess and stabilize patients with ACS. *Patients in this case have signs and symptoms of ACS, including possible AMI.* You will use the ACS Algorithm as the guide to clinical strategy.

The initial 12-lead ECG is used in all ACS cases to classify patients into 1 of 3 ECG categories, each with different strategies of care and management needs. These 3 ECG categories are ST-segment elevation suggesting ongoing acute injury, ST-segment depression suggesting ischemia, and nondiagnostic or normal ECG. These are outlined in the ACS Algorithm, but STEMI with time-sensitive reperfusion strategies is the focus of this course (Figure 20).

Key components of this case are

- Identification, assessment, and triage of acute ischemic chest discomfort
- Initial treatment of possible ACS
- Emphasis on early reperfusion of the patient with ACS/STEMI

Rhythms for ACS

Sudden cardiac death and hypotensive bradyarrhythmias may occur with acute ischemia. Providers will understand to anticipate these rhythms and be prepared for immediate attempts at defibrillation and administration of drug or electrical therapy for symptomatic bradyarrhythmias.

Although 12-lead ECG interpretation is beyond the scope of the ACLS Provider Course, some ACLS providers will have 12-lead ECG reading skills. For them, this case summarizes the identification and management of patients with STEMI.

Drugs for ACS

Drug therapy and treatment strategies continue to evolve rapidly in the field of ACS. ACLS providers and instructors will need to monitor important changes. The ACLS Provider Course presents only basic knowledge focusing on early treatment and the priority of rapid reperfusion, relief of ischemic pain, and treatment of early life-threatening complications. Reperfusion may involve the use of fibrinolytic therapy or coronary angiography with PCI (ie, balloon angioplasty/stenting). When used as the initial reperfusion strategy for STEMI, PCI is called *primary PCI*.

Treatment of ACS involves the initial use of drugs to relieve ischemic discomfort, dissolve clots, and inhibit thrombin and platelets. These drugs are

- Oxygen
- Aspirin
- Nitroglycerin
- Opiates (eg, morphine)
- Fibrinolytic therapy (overview)
- Heparin (UFH, LWMH)

Additional agents that are adjunctive to initial therapy and will not be discussed in the ACLS Provider Course are

- β-Blockers
- Adenosine diphosphate (ADP) antagonists (clopidogrel, prasugrel, ticagrelor)
- Angiotensin-converting enzyme (ACE) inhibitors
- HMG-CoA reductase inhibitors (statin therapy)
- Glycoprotein IIb/IIIa inhibitors

Goals for ACS Patients

OHCA Response

Half of the patients who die of ACS do so before reaching the hospital. VF or pulseless VT is the precipitating rhythm in most of these deaths. VF is most likely to develop during the first 4 hours after onset of symptoms.

Communities should develop programs to respond to OHCA. Such programs should focus on

- Recognizing symptoms of ACS
- Activating the EMS system, with EMS advance notification of the receiving hospital
- Providing early CPR
- Providing early defibrillation with AEDs available through public access defibrillation programs and first responders
- Providing a coordinated system of care among the EMS system, the ED, and Cardiology

The primary goals are

- Identification of patients with STEMI and triage for early reperfusion therapy
- Relief of ischemic chest discomfort
- Prevention of MACE, such as death, nonfatal MI, and the need for urgent postinfarction revascularization
- Treatment of acute, life-threatening complications of ACS, such as VF/pulseless VT, symptomatic bradycardias, and unstable tachycardias

Reperfusion therapy opens an occluded coronary artery with either mechanical means or drugs. PCI, performed in the heart catheterization suite after coronary angiography, allows balloon dilation and/or stent placement for an occluded coronary artery. "Clot-buster" drugs are called *fibrinolytics*, a more accurate term than *thrombolytics*.

Pathophysiology of ACS

Patients with coronary atherosclerosis may develop a spectrum of clinical syndromes representing varying degrees of coronary artery occlusion. These syndromes include non-ST elevation ACS (NSTE-ACS) and STEMI. Sudden cardiac death may occur with each of these syndromes. Figure 19 illustrates the pathophysiology of ACS.

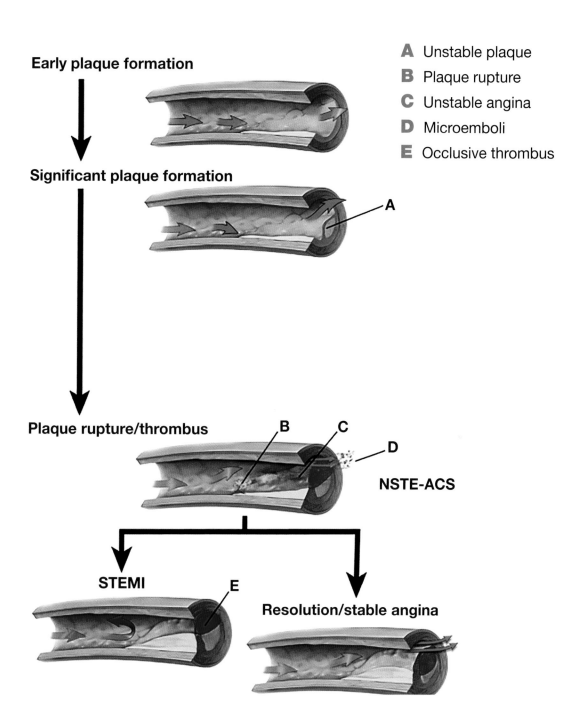

Figure 19. Pathophysiology of ACS.

Acute Coronary Syndromes Algorithm—2015 Update

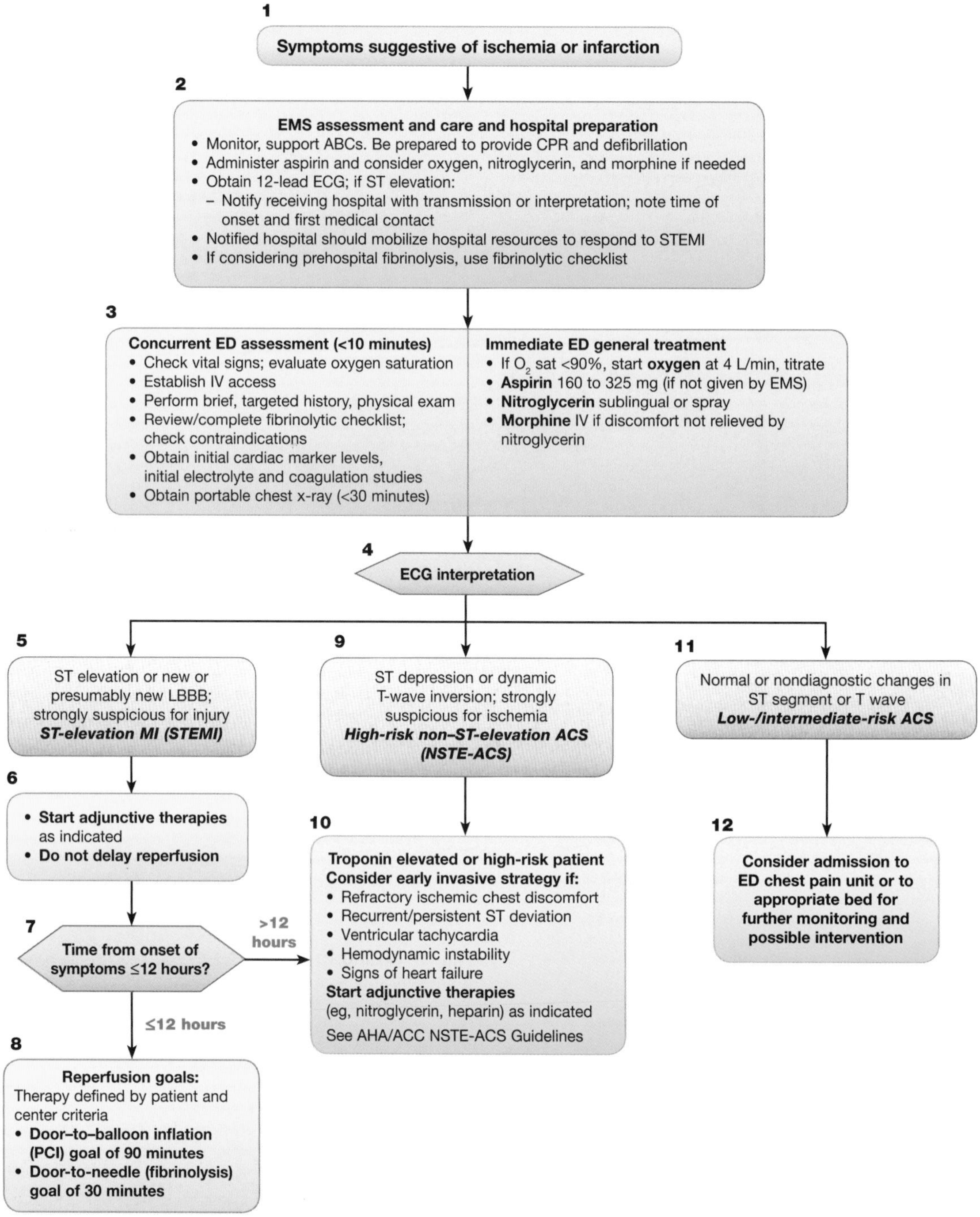

1
Symptoms suggestive of ischemia or infarction

2
EMS assessment and care and hospital preparation
- Monitor, support ABCs. Be prepared to provide CPR and defibrillation
- Administer aspirin and consider oxygen, nitroglycerin, and morphine if needed
- Obtain 12-lead ECG; if ST elevation:
  - Notify receiving hospital with transmission or interpretation; note time of onset and first medical contact
- Notified hospital should mobilize hospital resources to respond to STEMI
- If considering prehospital fibrinolysis, use fibrinolytic checklist

3
Concurrent ED assessment (<10 minutes)
- Check vital signs; evaluate oxygen saturation
- Establish IV access
- Perform brief, targeted history, physical exam
- Review/complete fibrinolytic checklist; check contraindications
- Obtain initial cardiac marker levels, initial electrolyte and coagulation studies
- Obtain portable chest x-ray (<30 minutes)

Immediate ED general treatment
- If O$_2$ sat <90%, start **oxygen** at 4 L/min, titrate
- **Aspirin** 160 to 325 mg (if not given by EMS)
- **Nitroglycerin** sublingual or spray
- **Morphine** IV if discomfort not relieved by nitroglycerin

4
ECG interpretation

5
ST elevation or new or presumably new LBBB; strongly suspicious for injury
ST-elevation MI (STEMI)

9
ST depression or dynamic T-wave inversion; strongly suspicious for ischemia
High-risk non–ST-elevation ACS (NSTE-ACS)

11
Normal or nondiagnostic changes in ST segment or T wave
Low-/intermediate-risk ACS

6
- Start adjunctive therapies as indicated
- Do not delay reperfusion

10
Troponin elevated or high-risk patient
Consider early invasive strategy if:
- Refractory ischemic chest discomfort
- Recurrent/persistent ST deviation
- Ventricular tachycardia
- Hemodynamic instability
- Signs of heart failure
Start adjunctive therapies
(eg, nitroglycerin, heparin) as indicated
See AHA/ACC NSTE-ACS Guidelines

12
Consider admission to ED chest pain unit or to appropriate bed for further monitoring and possible intervention

7
Time from onset of symptoms ≤12 hours?

>12 hours

≤12 hours

8
Reperfusion goals:
Therapy defined by patient and center criteria
- **Door–to–balloon inflation (PCI) goal of 90 minutes**
- **Door-to-needle (fibrinolysis) goal of 30 minutes**

© 2015 American Heart Association

Figure 20. The Acute Coronary Syndromes Algorithm.

Managing ACS: The Acute Coronary Syndromes Algorithm

Overview of the Algorithm

The Acute Coronary Syndromes Algorithm (Figure 20) outlines the assessment and management steps for a patient presenting with symptoms suggestive of ACS. The EMS responder in the out-of-hospital environment can begin immediate assessments and actions. These include giving oxygen, aspirin, nitroglycerin, and morphine if needed, and obtaining an initial 12-lead ECG (Step 2). Based on the ECG findings, the EMS provider may complete a fibrinolytic therapy checklist and notify the receiving ED of a potential

AMI-STEMI when appropriate (Step 3). If out-of-hospital providers are unable to complete these initial steps before the patient's arrival at the hospital, the ED provider should implement this component of care.

Subsequent treatment occurs on the patient's arrival at the hospital. ED personnel should review the out-of-hospital 12-lead ECG if available. If not performed, acquisition of the 12-lead ECG should be a priority. The goal is to analyze the 12-lead ECG as soon as possible within 10 minutes of the patient's arrival in the ED (Step 4). Hospital personnel should categorize patients into 1 of 3 groups according to analysis of the ST segment or the presence of left bundle branch block (LBBB) on the 12-lead ECG. Treatment recommendations are specific to each group.

- STEMI
- NSTE-ACS
- Low-/intermediate-risk ACS

The ACS Case will focus on the early reperfusion of the STEMI patient, emphasizing initial care and rapid triage for reperfusion therapy.

Important Considerations

The ACS Algorithm (Figure 20) provides general guidelines that apply to the initial triage of patients based on symptoms and the 12-lead ECG. Healthcare personnel often obtain serial cardiac markers (CK-MB, cardiac troponins) in most patients that allow additional risk stratification and treatment recommendations. Two important points for STEMI need emphasis:

- The ECG is central to the initial risk and treatment stratification process.
- Healthcare personnel do not need evidence of elevated cardiac markers to make a decision to administer fibrinolytic therapy or perform diagnostic coronary angiography with coronary intervention (angioplasty/stenting) in STEMI patients.

Application of the ACS Algorithm

The steps in the algorithm guide assessment and treatment:

- Identification of chest discomfort suggestive of ischemia (Step 1)
- EMS assessment, care, transport, and hospital prearrival notification (Step 2)
- Immediate ED assessment and treatment (Step 3)
- Classification of patients according to ST-segment analysis (Steps 5, 9, and 11)
- STEMI (Steps 5 through 8)

Identification of Chest Discomfort Suggestive of Ischemia

Signs and Conditions

You should know how to identify chest discomfort suggestive of ischemia. Conduct a prompt and targeted evaluation of every patient whose initial complaints suggest possible ACS.

The most common symptom of myocardial ischemia and infarction is retrosternal chest discomfort. The patient may perceive this discomfort more as pressure or tightness than actual pain.

Symptoms suggestive of ACS may also include

- Uncomfortable pressure, fullness, squeezing, or pain in the center of the chest lasting several minutes (usually more than a few minutes)
- Chest discomfort spreading to the shoulders, neck, one or both arms, or jaw
- Chest discomfort spreading into the back or between the shoulder blades
- Chest discomfort with light-headedness, dizziness, fainting, sweating, nausea, or vomiting
- Unexplained, sudden shortness of breath, which may occur with or without chest discomfort

Consider the likelihood that the presenting condition is ACS or one of its potentially lethal mimics. Other life-threatening conditions that may cause acute chest discomfort are aortic dissection, acute pulmonary embolism (PE), acute pericardial effusion with tamponade, and tension pneumothorax.

Foundational Facts

STEMI Chain of Survival

The STEMI Chain of Survival (Figure 21) described by the AHA is similar to the Chain of Survival for sudden cardiac arrest. It links actions to be taken by patients, family members, and healthcare providers to maximize STEMI recovery. These links are

- Rapid recognition and reaction to STEMI warning signs
- Rapid EMS dispatch and rapid EMS system transport and prearrival notification to the receiving hospital
- Rapid assessment and diagnosis in the ED (or cath lab)
- Rapid treatment

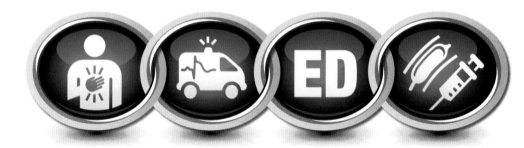

Figure 21. The STEMI Chain of Survival.

Starting With Dispatch

All dispatchers and EMS providers must receive training in ACS symptom recognition along with the potential complications. Dispatchers, when authorized by medical control or protocol, should tell patients with no history of aspirin allergy or signs of active or recent gastrointestinal (GI) bleeding to chew aspirin (160 to 325 mg) while waiting for EMS providers to arrive.

EMS Assessment, Care, and Hospital Preparation

Introduction

EMS assessment, care, and hospital preparation are outlined in Step 2. EMS responders may perform the following assessments and actions during the stabilization, triage, and transport of the patient to an appropriate facility:

- Monitor and support airway, breathing, and circulation (ABCs).
- Administer aspirin and consider oxygen if O_2 saturation is less than 90%, nitroglycerin, and morphine if discomfort is unresponsive to nitrates.
- Obtain a 12-lead ECG; interpret or transmit for interpretation.
- Complete a fibrinolytic checklist if indicated.
- Provide prearrival notification to the receiving facility if ST elevation.

Monitor and Support ABCs

Monitoring and support of ABCs includes

- Monitoring vital signs and cardiac rhythm
- Being prepared to provide CPR
- Using a defibrillator if needed

Administer Oxygen and Drugs

Providers should be familiar with the actions, indications, cautions, and treatment of side effects.

Oxygen

High inspired-oxygen tension will tend to maximize arterial oxygen saturation and, in turn, arterial oxygen content. This will help support oxygen delivery (cardiac output × arterial oxygen content) when cardiac output is limited. This short-term oxygen therapy does not produce oxygen toxicity.

EMS providers should administer **oxygen** if the patient is dyspneic, is hypoxemic, has obvious signs of heart failure, has an arterial oxygen saturation less than 90%, or the oxygen saturation is unknown. Providers should titrate oxygen therapy to a noninvasively monitored oxyhemoglobin saturation 90% or greater. Because its usefulness has not been established in normoxic patients with suspected or confirmed ACS, providers may consider withholding supplementary oxygen therapy in these patients.

Aspirin (Acetylsalicylic Acid)

A dose of 160 to 325 mg of non–enteric-coated aspirin causes immediate and near-total inhibition of thromboxane A_2 production by inhibiting platelet cyclooxygenase (COX-1). Platelets are one of the principal and earliest participants in thrombus formation. This rapid inhibition also reduces coronary reocclusion and other recurrent events independently and after fibrinolytic therapy.

If the patient has not taken **aspirin** and has no history of true aspirin allergy and no evidence of recent GI bleeding, give the patient aspirin (160 to 325 mg) to chew. In the initial hours of an ACS, aspirin is absorbed better when chewed than when swallowed, particularly if morphine has been given. Use rectal aspirin suppositories (300 mg) for patients with nausea, vomiting, active peptic ulcer disease, or other disorders of the upper GI tract.

Nitroglycerin (Glyceryl Trinitrate)

Nitroglycerin effectively reduces ischemic chest discomfort, and it has beneficial hemodynamic effects. The physiologic effects of nitrates cause reduction in LV and right ventricular (RV) preload through peripheral arterial and venous dilation.

Give the patient 1 sublingual **nitroglycerin** tablet (or spray "dose") every 3 to 5 minutes for ongoing symptoms if it is permitted by medical control and no contraindications exist. Healthcare providers may repeat the dose twice (total of 3 doses). Administer nitroglycerin only if the patient remains hemodynamically stable: SBP is greater than 90 mm Hg or no lower than 30 mm Hg below baseline (if known) and the heart rate is 50 to 100/min.

Nitroglycerin is a venodilator and needs to be used cautiously or not at all in patients with inadequate ventricular preload. These situations include

- **Inferior wall MI and RV infarction.** RV infarction may complicate an inferior wall MI. Patients with acute RV infarction are very dependent on RV filling pressures to maintain cardiac output and blood pressure. If RV infarction cannot be ruled out, providers must use caution in administering nitrates to patients with inferior STEMI. If RV infarction is confirmed by right-sided precordial leads or clinical findings by an experienced provider, nitroglycerin and other vasodilators (morphine) or volume-depleting drugs (diuretics) are contraindicated as well.
- **Hypotension, bradycardia, or tachycardia.** Avoid use of nitroglycerin in patients with hypotension (SBP less than 90 mm Hg), marked bradycardia (less than 50/min), or tachycardia.
- **Recent phosphodiesterase inhibitor use.** Avoid the use of nitroglycerin if it is suspected or known that the patient has taken sildenafil or vardenafil within the previous 24 hours or tadalafil within 48 hours. These agents are generally used for erectile dysfunction or in cases of pulmonary hypertension and in combination with nitrates may cause severe hypotension refractory to vasopressor agents.

Opiates (eg, Morphine)

Give an opiate (eg, *morphine)* for chest discomfort unresponsive to sublingual or spray nitroglycerin if authorized by protocol or medical control. Morphine is indicated in STEMI when chest discomfort is unresponsive to nitrates. Use morphine with caution in NSTE-ACS because of an association with increased mortality.

Morphine may be utilized in the management of ACS because it

- Produces central nervous system analgesia, which reduces the adverse effects of neurohumoral activation, catecholamine release, and heightened myocardial oxygen demand
- Produces venodilation, which reduces LV preload and oxygen requirements
- Decreases systemic vascular resistance, thereby reducing LV afterload
- Helps redistribute blood volume in patients with acute pulmonary edema

Remember, morphine is a venodilator. Like nitroglycerin, use smaller doses and carefully monitor physiologic response before administering additional doses in patients who may be preload dependent. If hypotension develops, administer fluids as a first line of therapy.

Critical Concepts

Pain Relief With Nitroglycerin

Relief of pain with nitroglycerin is neither specific nor a useful diagnostic tool to determine the etiology of symptoms in ED patients with chest pain or discomfort. GI etiologies as well as other causes of chest discomfort can "respond" to nitroglycerin administration. Therefore, the response to nitrate therapy is not diagnostic of ACS.

Caution

Use of Nonsteroidal Anti-inflammatory Drugs

Use of nonsteroidal anti-inflammatory drugs (NSAIDs) is contraindicated (except for aspirin) and should be discontinued. Both nonselective as well as COX-2 selective drugs should not be administered during hospitalization for STEMI because of the increased risk of mortality, reinfarction, hypertension, heart failure, and myocardial rupture associated with their use.

Obtain a 12-Lead ECG

EMS providers should obtain a 12-lead ECG. The AHA recommends out-of-hospital 12-lead ECG diagnostic programs in urban and suburban EMS systems.

EMS Action	Recommendation
12-Lead ECG if available	The AHA recommends routine use of 12-lead out-of-hospital ECGs for patients with signs and symptoms of possible ACS.
Prearrival hospital notification for STEMI	Prearrival notification of the ED shortens the time to treatment (10 to 60 minutes has been achieved in clinical studies) and speeds reperfusion therapy with fibrinolytics or PCI or both, which may reduce mortality and minimize myocardial injury.
Fibrinolytic checklist if appropriate	If STEMI is identified on the 12-lead ECG, complete a fibrinolytic checklist if appropriate.

 See the Student Website (**www.heart.org/eccstudent**) for a sample fibrinolytic checklist.

Immediate ED Assessment and Treatment

Introduction

The high-performance team should quickly evaluate the patient with potential ACS on the patient's arrival in the ED. Within the first 10 minutes, obtain a 12-lead ECG (if not already performed before arrival) and assess the patient.

The 12-lead ECG (example in Figure 22) is at the center of the decision pathway in the management of ischemic chest discomfort and is the only means of identifying STEMI.

A targeted evaluation should be performed and focus on chest discomfort, signs and symptoms of heart failure, cardiac history, risk factors for ACS, and historical features that may preclude the use of fibrinolytics. For the patient with STEMI, the goals of reperfusion are to give fibrinolytics within 30 minutes of arrival or perform PCI within 90 minutes of arrival.

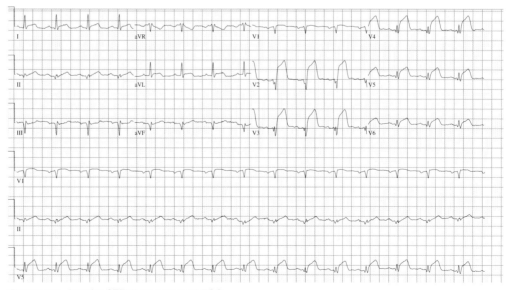

Figure 22. Anterior STEMI on a 12-lead ECG.

Figure 23 shows how to measure ST-segment deviation.

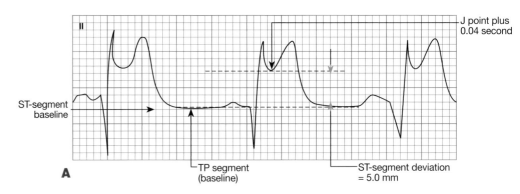

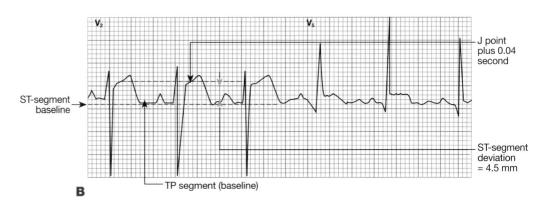

Figure 23. How to measure ST-segment deviation. **A,** Inferior MI. The ST segment has no low point (it is covered or concave). **B,** Anterior MI.

The First 10 Minutes

Assessment and stabilization of the patient in the first 10 minutes should include the following:

- Check vital signs and evaluate oxygen saturation.
- Establish IV access.
- Take a brief focused history and perform a physical examination.
- Complete the fibrinolytic checklist and check for contraindications, if indicated.
- Obtain a blood sample to evaluate initial cardiac marker levels, electrolytes, and coagulation.
- Obtain and review portable chest x-ray (less than 30 minutes after the patient's arrival in the ED). This should not delay fibrinolytic therapy for STEMI or activation of the PCI team for STEMI.

Note: The results of cardiac markers, chest x-ray, and laboratory studies should not delay reperfusion therapy unless clinically necessary, eg, suspected aortic dissection or coagulopathy.

Patient General Treatment

Unless allergies or contraindications exist, 4 agents may be considered in patients with ischemic-type chest discomfort:

- Oxygen if hypoxemic (O_2 % less than 90%) or signs of heart failure
- Aspirin
- Nitroglycerin
- Opiate (eg, morphine if ongoing discomfort or no response to nitrates)

Because these agents may have been given out of hospital, administer initial or supplementary doses as indicated. (See the discussion of these drugs in the previous section, EMS Assessment, Care, and Hospital Preparation.)

Critical Concepts

Oxygen, Aspirin, Nitrates, and Opiates

- Unless contraindicated, initial therapy with oxygen if needed, aspirin, nitrates, and, if indicated, morphine is recommended for all patients suspected of having ischemic chest discomfort.
- The major contraindication to nitroglycerin and morphine is hypotension, including hypotension from an RV infarction. The major contraindications to aspirin are true aspirin allergy and active or recent GI bleeding.

Classify Patients According to ST-Segment Deviation

Classify Into 3 Groups Based on ST-Segment Deviation

Review the initial 12-lead ECG (Step 4) and classify patients into 1 of the 3 following clinical groups (Steps 5, 9, and 11):

General Group	Description
STEMI	ST elevation
NSTE-ACS	ST depression or dynamic T-wave inversion
Low-/intermediate-risk ACS	Normal or nondiagnostic ECG

- **STEMI** is characterized by ST-segment elevation in 2 or more contiguous leads or new LBBB. Threshold values for ST-segment elevation consistent with STEMI are J-point elevation greater than 2 mm (0.2 mV) in leads V_2 and V_3* and 1 mm or more in all other leads or by new or presumed new LBBB.
  *2.5 mm in men younger than 40 years; 1.5 mm in all women.
- **NSTE-ACS** is characterized by ischemic ST-segment depression 0.5 mm (0.05 mV) or greater or dynamic T-wave inversion with pain or discomfort. Nonpersistent or transient ST elevation 0.5 mm or greater for less than 20 minutes is also included in this category.
- **Low-/intermediate-risk ACS** is characterized by normal or nondiagnostic changes in the ST segment or T wave that are inconclusive and require further risk stratification. This classification includes patients with normal ECGs and those with ST-segment deviation in either direction of less than 0.5 mm (0.05 mV) or T-wave inversion ≤2 mm or 0.2 mV. Serial cardiac studies and functional testing are appropriate. Note that additional information (troponin) may place the patient into a higher risk classification after initial classification.

The ECG classification of ischemic syndromes is not meant to be exclusive. A small percentage of patients with normal ECGs may be found to have MI, for example. If the initial ECG is nondiagnostic and clinical circumstances indicate (eg, ongoing chest discomfort), repeat the ECG.

STEMI

Introduction

Patients with STEMI usually have complete occlusion of an epicardial coronary artery.

The mainstay of treatment for STEMI is early reperfusion therapy achieved with primary PCI or fibrinolytics.

Reperfusion therapy for STEMI is perhaps the most important advancement in treatment of cardiovascular disease in recent years. Early fibrinolytic therapy or direct catheter-based reperfusion has been established as a standard of care for patients with STEMI who present within 12 hours of onset of symptoms with no contraindications. Reperfusion therapy reduces mortality and saves heart muscle; the shorter the time to reperfusion, the greater the benefit. A 47% reduction in mortality was noted when fibrinolytic therapy was provided in the first hour after onset of symptoms.

Critical Concepts

Delay of Therapy

- Routine consultation with a cardiologist or another physician should not delay diagnosis and treatment except in equivocal or uncertain cases. Consultation delays therapy and is associated with increased hospital mortality rates.
- Potential delay during the in-hospital evaluation period may occur from **door** to data (ECG), from **data** to decision, and from **decision** to **drug** (or PCI). These 4 major points of in-hospital therapy are commonly referred to as the "4 D's."
- All providers must focus on minimizing delays at each of these points. Out-of-hospital transport time constitutes only 5% of delay to treatment time; ED evaluation constitutes 25% to 33% of this delay.

Early Reperfusion Therapy

Rapidly identify patients with STEMI and quickly screen them for indications and contraindications to fibrinolytic therapy by using a fibrinolytic checklist if appropriate.

The first qualified physician who encounters a patient with STEMI should interpret or confirm the 12-lead ECG, determine the risk/benefit of reperfusion therapy, and direct administration of fibrinolytic therapy or activation of the PCI team. Early activation of PCI may occur with established protocols. The following time frames are recommended:

- For *PCI,* this goal for ED door–to–balloon inflation time is 90 minutes. In patients presenting to a non–PCI-capable hospital, time from first medical contact to device should be less than 120 minutes when primary PCI is considered.
- If fibrinolysis is the intended reperfusion, an ED door-to-needle time (needle time is the beginning of infusion of a fibrinolytic agent) of 30 minutes is the medical system goal that is considered the longest time acceptable. Systems should strive to achieve the shortest time possible.
- Patients who are ineligible for *fibrinolytic therapy* should be considered for transfer to a PCI facility regardless of delay. The system should prepare for a door-to-departure time of 30 minutes when a transfer decision is made.

Adjunctive treatments may also be indicated.

Use of PCI

The most commonly used form of PCI is coronary intervention with stent placement. Optimally performed *primary PCI* is the preferred reperfusion strategy over fibrinolytic administration. *Rescue PCI* is used early after fibrinolytics in patients who may have persistent occlusion of the infarct artery (failure to reperfuse with fibrinolytics), although this term has been recently replaced and included by the term *pharmacoinvasive strategy*. PCI has been shown to be superior to fibrinolysis in the combined end points of death, stroke, and reinfarction in many studies for patients presenting between 3 and 12 hours after onset. However, these results have been achieved in experienced medical settings with skilled providers (performing more than 75 PCIs per year) at a skilled PCI facility (performing more than 200 PCIs for STEMI with cardiac surgery capabilities).

Considerations for the use of PCI include the following:

- PCI is the treatment of choice for the management of STEMI when it can be performed effectively with a door-to-balloon time of less than 90 minutes from first medical contact by a skilled provider at a skilled PCI facility.
- Primary PCI may also be offered to patients presenting to non–PCI-capable centers if PCI can be initiated promptly within 120 minutes from first medical contact. The TRANSFER AMI (Trial of Routine Angioplasty and Stenting After Fibrinolysis to Enhance Reperfusion in Acute Myocardial Infarction) trial supports the transfer of high-risk patients who receive fibrinolysis in a non-PCI center within 12 hours of symptom onset to a PCI center within 6 hours of fibrinolytic administration to receive routine early coronary angiography and PCI if indicated.
- For patients admitted to a hospital without PCI capabilities, there may be some benefit associated with transfer for PCI versus administration of on-site fibrinolytics in terms of reinfarction, stroke, and a trend to lower mortality when PCI can be performed within 120 minutes of first medical contact.
- PCI is also preferred in patients with contraindications to fibrinolytics and is indicated in patients with cardiogenic shock or heart failure complicating MI..

Use of Fibrinolytic Therapy

A fibrinolytic agent or "clot-buster" is administered to patients with J-point ST-segment elevation greater than 2 mm (0.2 mV) in leads V_2 and V_3 and 1 mm or more in all other leads or by new or presumed new LBBB (eg, leads III, aVF; leads V_3, V_4; leads I and aVL) without contraindications. Fibrin-specific agents are effective in achieving normal flow in about 50% of patients given these drugs. Examples of fibrin-specific drugs are rtPA, reteplase, and tenecteplase. Streptokinase was the first fibrinolytic used widely, but it is not fibrin specific.

Considerations for the use of fibrinolytic therapy are as follows:

- In the absence of contraindications and in the presence of a favorable risk-benefit ratio, fibrinolytic therapy is one option for reperfusion in patients with STEMI and *onset of symptoms within 12 hours of presentation* with qualifying ECG findings and if PCI is not available within 90 minutes of first medical contact.
- In the absence of contraindications, it is also reasonable to give fibrinolytics to patients with *onset of symptoms within the prior 12 hours* and ECG findings consistent with true posterior MI. Experienced providers will recognize this as a condition where ST-segment depression in the early precordial leads is equivalent to ST-segment elevation in others. When these changes are associated with other ECG findings, it is suggestive of a "STEMI" on the posterior wall of the heart.
- Fibrinolytics are generally not recommended for patients presenting *more than 12 hours after onset of symptoms*. But they may be considered if ischemic chest discomfort continues with persistent ST-segment elevation.
- Do not give fibrinolytics to patients who present *more than 24 hours after the onset of symptoms* or patients with ST-segment depression unless a true posterior MI is suspected.

Adjunctive Treatments

Other drugs are useful when indicated in addition to oxygen, sublingual or spray nitroglycerin, aspirin, morphine, and fibrinolytic therapy. These include

- Unfractionated or low-molecular-weight heparin
- Bivalirudin
- P2Y$_{12}$ inhibitors
- IV nitroglycerin
- β-Blockers
- Glycoprotein IIb/IIIa inhibitors

IV nitroglycerin and heparin are commonly used early in the management of patients with STEMI. These agents are briefly discussed below. Use of bivalirudin, P2Y$_{12}$ inhibitors, β-blockers, and glycoprotein IIb/IIIa inhibitors will not be reviewed. Use of these agents requires additional risk stratification skills and a detailed knowledge of the spectrum of ACS and, in some instances, continuing knowledge of the results of clinical trials.

Heparin (Unfractionated or Low-Molecular-Weight)

Heparin is routinely given as an adjunct for PCI and fibrinolytic therapy with fibrin-specific agents (rtPA, reteplase, tenecteplase). It is also indicated in other specific high-risk situations, such as LV mural thrombus, atrial fibrillation, and prophylaxis for venous thrombo-embolism in patients with prolonged bed rest and heart failure complicating MI. If you use these drugs, you must be familiar with dosing schedules for specific clinical strategies.

The inappropriate dosing and monitoring of heparin therapy has caused excess intracerebral bleeding and major hemorrhage in STEMI patients. Providers using heparin need to know the indications, dosing, and use in the specific ACS categories.

The dosing, use, and duration have been derived from use in clinical trials. Specific patients may require dose modification. See the ECC Handbook for weight-based dosing guidelines, intervals of administration, and adjustment of low-molecular-weight heparin in renal function. See the ACC/AHA guidelines for detailed discussion in specific categories.

IV Nitroglycerin

Routine use of IV nitroglycerin is not indicated and has not been shown to significantly reduce mortality in STEMI. IV nitroglycerin is indicated and used widely in ischemic syndromes. It is preferred over topical or long-acting forms because it can be titrated in a patient with potentially unstable hemodynamics and clinical condition. Indications for initiation of IV nitroglycerin in STEMI are

- Recurrent or continuing chest discomfort unresponsive to sublingual or spray nitroglycerin
- Pulmonary edema complicating STEMI
- Hypertension complicating STEMI

Treatment goals using IV nitroglycerin are as follows:

Treatment Goal	Management
Relief of ischemic chest discomfort	• Titrate to effect • Keep SBP greater than 90 mm Hg • Limit drop in SBP to 30 mm Hg below baseline in hypertensive patients
Improvement in pulmonary edema and hypertension	• Titrate to effect • Limit drop in SBP to 10% of baseline in normotensive patients • Limit drop in SBP to 30 mm Hg below baseline in hypertensive patients

Acute Stroke Case

Introduction

The identification and initial management of patients with acute stroke is within the scope of an ACLS provider. This case covers *principles of out-of-hospital care* and *fundamental aspects of initial in-hospital acute stroke care.*

Out-of-hospital acute stroke care focuses on

- Rapid identification and assessment of patients with stroke
- Rapid transport (with prearrival notification) to a facility capable of providing acute stroke care

In-hospital acute stroke care includes the

- Ability to rapidly determine patient eligibility for fibrinolytic therapy
- Administration of fibrinolytic therapy to appropriate candidates, with availability of neurologic medical supervision within target times
- Consideration of new treatment options like endovascular therapy
- Initiation of the stroke pathway and patient admission to a stroke unit if available

The target times and goals are recommended by the NINDS, which has recommended measurable goals for the evaluation of stroke patients. These targets or goals should be achieved for at least 80% of patients with acute stroke.

Potential Arrhythmias With Stroke

The ECG does not take priority over obtaining a computed tomography (CT) scan. No arrhythmias are specific for stroke, but the ECG may identify evidence of a recent AMI or arrhythmias such as atrial fibrillation as a cause of an embolic stroke. Many patients with stroke may demonstrate arrhythmias, but if the patient is hemodynamically stable, most arrhythmias will not require treatment. There is general agreement to recommend cardiac monitoring during the first 24 hours of evaluation in patients with acute ischemic stroke to detect atrial fibrillation and potentially life-threatening arrhythmias.

Drugs for Stroke

This case involves these drugs:

- Approved fibrinolytic agent (rtPA)
- Glucose (D_{50})
- Labetalol
- Nicardipine
- Enalaprilat
- Aspirin
- Nitroprusside

Major Types of Stroke

Stroke is a general term. It refers to acute neurologic impairment that follows interruption in blood supply to a specific area of the brain. Although expeditious stroke care is important for all patients, this case emphasizes reperfusion therapy for acute ischemic stroke.

The major types of stroke are

- Ischemic stroke: Accounts for 87% of all strokes and is usually caused by an occlusion of an artery to a region of the brain (Figure 24).
- Hemorrhagic stroke: Accounts for 13% of all strokes and occurs when a blood vessel in the brain suddenly ruptures into the surrounding tissue. Fibrinolytic therapy is contraindicated in this type of stroke. Avoid anticoagulants.

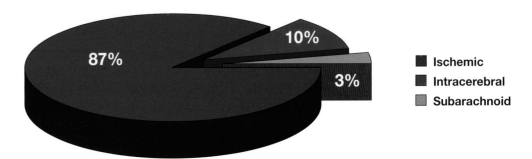

Figure 24. Types of stroke. Eighty-seven percent of strokes are ischemic and potentially eligible for fibrinolytic therapy if patients otherwise qualify. Thirteen percent of strokes are hemorrhagic, and the majority of these are intracerebral. The male-to-female incidence ratio is 1.25 in persons 55 to 64 years of age, 1.50 in those 65 to 74, 1.07 in those 75 to 84, and 0.76 in those 85 and older. Blacks have almost twice the risk of first-ever stroke compared with whites.

Approach to Stroke Care

Introduction

Each year in the United States, about 795 000 people have a new or recurrent stroke. Stroke remains a leading cause of death in the United States.

Early recognition of acute ischemic stroke is important because IV fibrinolytic treatment should be provided as early as possible, generally within 3 hours of onset of symptoms, or within 4.5 hours of onset of symptoms for selected patients. Endovascular therapy may be given within 6 hours of onset of symptoms, but better outcomes are associated with shorter times to treatment. Most strokes occur at home, and only half of acute stroke patients use EMS for transport to the hospital. Stroke patients often deny or try to rationalize their symptoms. Even high-risk patients, such as those with atrial fibrillation or hypertension, fail to recognize the signs of stroke. This delays activation of EMS and treatment, resulting in increased morbidity and mortality.

Community and professional education is essential, and it has been successful in increasing the proportion of eligible stroke patients treated with fibrinolytic therapy. Healthcare providers, hospitals, and communities must continue to develop systems to improve the efficiency and effectiveness of stroke care.

Foundational Facts

Stroke Chain of Survival

The goal of stroke care is to minimize brain injury and maximize the patient's recovery. The Stroke Chain of Survival (Figure 25) described by the AHA and the American Stroke Association is similar to the Chain of Survival for sudden cardiac arrest. It links actions to be taken by patients, family members, and healthcare providers to maximize stroke recovery. These links are

- Rapid recognition and reaction to stroke warning signs
- Rapid EMS dispatch
- Rapid EMS system transport and prearrival notification to the receiving hospital
- Rapid diagnosis and treatment in the hospital

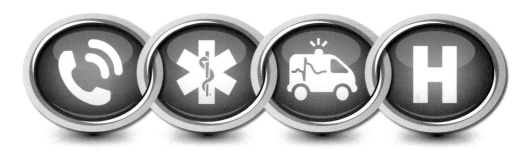

Figure 25. The Stroke Chain of Survival.

Foundational Facts

The 8 D's of Stroke Care

The 8 D's of Stroke Care highlight the major steps in diagnosis and treatment of stroke and key points at which delays can occur:

- **Detection:** Rapid recognition of stroke symptoms
- **Dispatch:** Early activation and dispatch of EMS by 9-1-1
- **Delivery:** Rapid EMS identification, management, and transport
- **Door:** Appropriate triage to stroke center
- **Data:** Rapid triage, evaluation, and management within the ED
- **Decision:** Stroke expertise and therapy selection
- **Drug/Device:** Fibrinolytic or endovascular therapy
- **Disposition:** Rapid admission to the stroke unit or critical care unit

For more information on these critical elements, see the Adult Suspected Stroke Algorithm (Figure 26).

Goals of Stroke Care

The Suspected Stroke Algorithm (Figure 26) emphasizes important elements of out-of-hospital care for possible stroke patients. These actions include a stroke scale or screen and rapid transport to the hospital. As with ACS, prior notification of the receiving hospital speeds the care of the stroke patient upon arrival.

The NINDS has established critical in-hospital time goals for assessment and management of patients with suspected stroke. This algorithm reviews the critical in-hospital time periods for patient assessment and treatment:

1. Immediate general assessment by the stroke team, emergency physician, or another expert within *10 minutes* of arrival; order urgent noncontrast CT scan

2. Neurologic assessment by the stroke team or designee and CT scan performed within *25 minutes* of hospital arrival

3. Interpretation of the CT scan within *45 minutes* of ED arrival

4. Initiation of fibrinolytic therapy in appropriate patients (those without contraindications) within *1 hour* of hospital arrival and *3 hours* from symptom onset

5. Door-to-admission time of *3 hours*

Foundational Facts

The National Institute of Neurological Disorders and Stroke

The NINDS is a branch of the National Institutes of Health (NIH). Its mission is to reduce the burden of neurologic disease by supporting and conducting research. NINDS researchers have studied stroke and reviewed data leading to recommendations for acute stroke care. The NINDS has set critical time goals for assessment and management of stroke patients based on experience obtained in large studies of stroke patients.

Critical Time Periods

Patients with acute ischemic stroke have a time-dependent benefit for fibrinolytic therapy similar to that of patients with ST-segment elevation MI, but this time-dependent benefit is much shorter.

The critical time period for administration of *IV* fibrinolytic therapy begins with the onset of symptoms. Critical time periods from hospital arrival are summarized below:

Immediate general assessment	10 minutes
Immediate neurologic assessment	25 minutes
Acquisition of CT of the head	25 minutes
Interpretation of the CT scan	45 minutes
Administration of fibrinolytic therapy, timed from ED arrival	60 minutes
Administration of fibrinolytic therapy, timed from onset of symptoms	3 hours, or 4.5 hours in selected patients
Administration of endovascular therapy, timed from onset of symptoms	6 hours in selected patients
Admission to a monitored bed	3 hours

Adult Suspected Stroke Algorithm

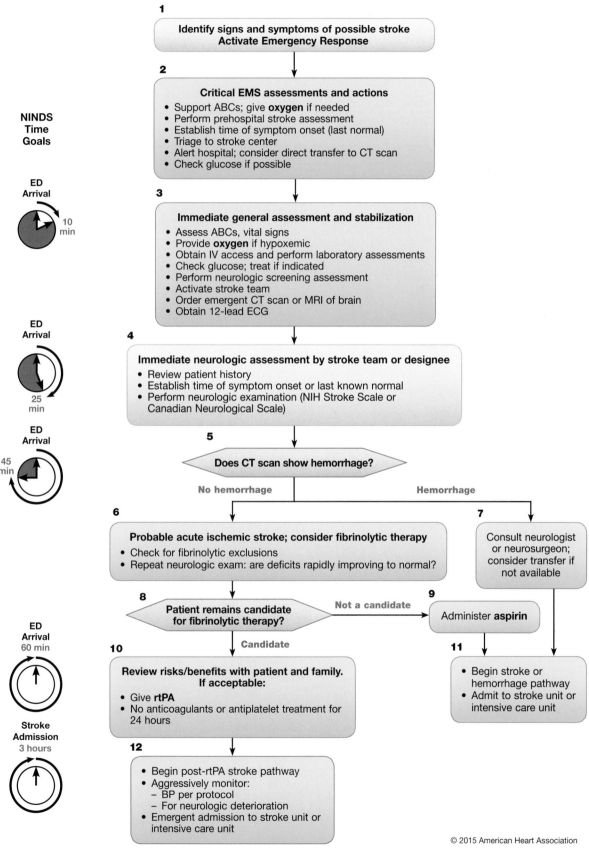

NINDS Time Goals

ED Arrival — 10 min

ED Arrival — 25 min

ED Arrival — 45 min

ED Arrival 60 min

Stroke Admission 3 hours

1
Identify signs and symptoms of possible stroke
Activate Emergency Response

2
Critical EMS assessments and actions
- Support ABCs; give **oxygen** if needed
- Perform prehospital stroke assessment
- Establish time of symptom onset (last normal)
- Triage to stroke center
- Alert hospital; consider direct transfer to CT scan
- Check glucose if possible

3
Immediate general assessment and stabilization
- Assess ABCs, vital signs
- Provide **oxygen** if hypoxemic
- Obtain IV access and perform laboratory assessments
- Check glucose; treat if indicated
- Perform neurologic screening assessment
- Activate stroke team
- Order emergent CT scan or MRI of brain
- Obtain 12-lead ECG

4
Immediate neurologic assessment by stroke team or designee
- Review patient history
- Establish time of symptom onset or last known normal
- Perform neurologic examination (NIH Stroke Scale or Canadian Neurological Scale)

5
Does CT scan show hemorrhage?

No hemorrhage / Hemorrhage

6
Probable acute ischemic stroke; consider fibrinolytic therapy
- Check for fibrinolytic exclusions
- Repeat neurologic exam: are deficits rapidly improving to normal?

7
Consult neurologist or neurosurgeon; consider transfer if not available

8
Patient remains candidate for fibrinolytic therapy?

Not a candidate → / Candidate

9
Administer **aspirin**

10
Review risks/benefits with patient and family. If acceptable:
- Give **rtPA**
- No anticoagulants or antiplatelet treatment for 24 hours

11
- Begin stroke or hemorrhage pathway
- Admit to stroke unit or intensive care unit

12
- Begin post-rtPA stroke pathway
- Aggressively monitor:
  – BP per protocol
  – For neurologic deterioration
- Emergent admission to stroke unit or intensive care unit

© 2015 American Heart Association

Figure 26. The Adult Suspected Stroke Algorithm.

Application of the Suspected Stroke Algorithm

We will now discuss the steps in the algorithm, as well as other related topics:

- Identification of signs and symptoms of possible stroke and activation of emergency response (Step 1)
- Critical EMS assessments and actions (Step 2)
- Immediate general assessment and stabilization (Step 3)
- Immediate neurologic assessment by the stroke team or designee (Step 4)
- CT scan: hemorrhage or no hemorrhage (Step 5)
- Fibrinolytic therapy risk stratification if candidate (Steps 6, 8, and 10)
- General stroke care (Steps 11 and 12)

Identification of Signs of Possible Stroke

Warning Signs and Symptoms

The signs and symptoms of a stroke may be subtle. They include

- Sudden weakness or numbness of the face, arm, or leg, especially on one side of the body
- Sudden confusion
- Trouble speaking or understanding
- Sudden trouble seeing in one or both eyes
- Sudden trouble walking
- Dizziness or loss of balance or coordination
- Sudden severe headache with no known cause

Activate EMS System Immediately

Stroke patients and their families must be educated to activate EMS as soon as they detect potential signs or symptoms of stroke. Currently half of all stroke patients are driven to the ED by family or friends.

EMS provides the safest and most efficient method of emergency transport to the hospital. The advantages of EMS transport include the following:

- EMS personnel can identify and transport a stroke patient to a hospital capable of providing acute stroke care and notify the hospital of the patient's impending arrival.
- Prearrival notification allows the hospital to prepare to evaluate and manage the patient efficiently.

Emergency medical dispatchers also play a critical role in timely treatment of potential stroke by

- Identifying possible stroke patients
- Providing high-priority dispatch
- Instructing bystanders in lifesaving CPR skills or other supportive care if needed while EMS providers are on the way

Stroke Assessment Tools

The AHA recommends that all EMS personnel be trained to recognize stroke by using a validated, abbreviated out-of-hospital neurologic evaluation tool such as the Cincinnati Prehospital Stroke Scale (CPSS) (Table 5).

Cincinnati Prehospital Stroke Scale

The CPSS identifies stroke on the basis of 3 physical findings:

- Facial droop (have the patient smile or try to show teeth)
- Arm drift (have the patient close eyes and hold both arms out, with palms up)
- Abnormal speech (have the patient say, "You can't teach an old dog new tricks")

By using the CPSS, medical personnel can evaluate the patient in less than 1 minute. The presence of 1 finding on the CPSS has a sensitivity of 59% and a specificity of 89% when scored by prehospital providers.

With standard training in stroke recognition, paramedics demonstrated a sensitivity of 61% to 66% for identifying patients with stroke. After receiving training in use of a stroke assessment tool, paramedic sensitivity for identifying patients with stroke increased to 86% to 97%.

Table 5. The Cincinnati Prehospital Stroke Scale

Test	Findings
Facial droop: Have the patient show teeth or smile (Figure 27)	**Normal**—both sides of face move equally **Abnormal**—one side of face does not move as well as the other side
Arm drift: Patient closes eyes and extends both arms straight out, with palms up, for 10 seconds (Figure 28)	**Normal**—both arms move the same *or* both arms do not move at all (other findings, such as pronator drift, may be helpful) **Abnormal**—one arm does not move *or* one arm drifts down compared with the other
Abnormal speech: Have patient say, "you can't teach an old dog new tricks"	**Normal**—patient uses correct words with no slurring **Abnormal**—patient slurs words, uses the wrong words, or is unable to speak

Interpretation: If any 1 of these 3 signs is abnormal, the probability of a stroke is 72%. The presence of all 3 findings indicates that the probability of stroke is greater than 85%.

Modified from Kothari RU, Pancioli A, Liu T, Brott T, Broderick J. Cincinnati Prehospital Stroke Scale: reproducibility and validity. *Ann Emerg Med.* 1999;33(4):373-378. With permission from Elsevier.

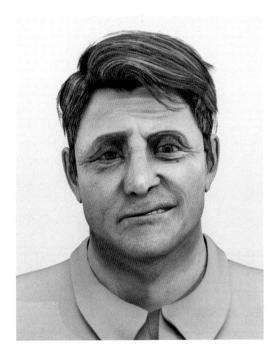

Figure 27. Facial droop.

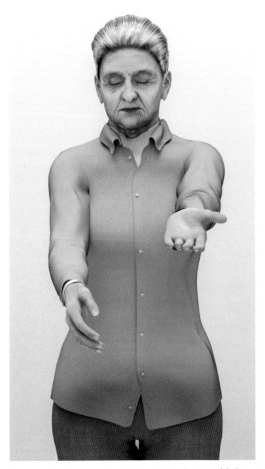

Figure 28. One-sided motor weakness (right arm).

Critical EMS Assessments and Actions

Introduction

Prehospital EMS providers must minimize the interval between the onset of symptoms and patient arrival in the ED. Specific stroke therapy can be provided only in the appropriate receiving hospital ED, so time in the field only delays (and may prevent) definitive therapy. More extensive assessments and initiation of supportive therapies can continue en route to the hospital or in the ED.

Critical EMS Assessments and Actions

To provide the best outcome for the patient with potential stroke, do the following:

Identify Signs	Define and Recognize the Signs of Stroke (Step 1)
Support ABCs	Support the ABCs and provide supplementary oxygen to hypoxemic (eg, oxygen saturation less than 94%) stroke patients or those patients with unknown oxygen saturation.
Perform stroke assessment	Perform a rapid out-of-hospital stroke assessment (CPSS, Table 5).
Establish time	Determine when the patient was last known to be normal or at neurologic baseline. This represents time zero. If the patient wakes from sleep with symptoms of stroke, time zero is the last time the patient was seen to be normal.
Triage to stroke center	Transport the patient rapidly and consider triage to a stroke center. Support cardiopulmonary function during transport. If possible, bring a witness, family member, or caregiver with the patient to confirm time of onset of stroke symptoms.
Alert hospital	Provide prearrival notification to the receiving hospital.
Check glucose	During transport, check blood glucose if protocols or medical control allows.

The patient with acute stroke is at risk for respiratory compromise from aspiration, upper airway obstruction, hypoventilation, and (rarely) neurogenic pulmonary edema. The combination of poor perfusion and hypoxemia will exacerbate and extend ischemic brain injury, and it has been associated with worse outcome from stroke.

Both out-of-hospital and in-hospital medical personnel should provide supplementary oxygen to hypoxemic (ie, oxygen saturation less than 94%) stroke patients or patients for whom oxygen saturation is unknown.

Foundational Facts

Stroke Centers and Stroke Units

Initial evidence indicates a favorable benefit from triage of stroke patients directly to designated stroke centers, but the concept of routine out-of-hospital triage of stroke patients requires continued evaluation.

Each receiving hospital should define its capability for treating patients with acute stroke and should communicate this information to the EMS system and the community. Although not every hospital has the resources to safely administer fibrinolytics or endovascular therapy, every hospital with an ED should have a written plan that describes how patients with acute stroke will be managed in that institution. The plan should

- Detail the roles of healthcare providers in the care of patients with acute stroke, including identifying sources of neurologic expertise
- Define which patients to treat with fibrinolytics or endovascular therapy at that facility
- Describe when patient transfer to another hospital with a dedicated stroke unit is appropriate

Patients with stroke should be admitted to a stroke unit when a stroke unit with a multidisciplinary team experienced in managing stroke is available within a reasonable transport interval.

Studies have documented improvement in 1-year survival rate, functional outcomes, and quality of life when patients hospitalized for acute stroke receive care in a dedicated unit with a specialized team.

In-Hospital, Immediate General Assessment and Stabilization

Introduction

Once the patient arrives in the ED, a number of assessments and management activities must occur quickly. Protocols should be used to minimize delay in definitive diagnosis and therapy.

The goal of the stroke team, emergency physician, or other experts should be to assess the patient with suspected stroke within 10 minutes of arrival in the ED: "time is brain" (Step 3).

Immediate General Assessment and Stabilization

ED providers should do the following:

Step	Actions
Assess ABCs	Assess the ABCs and evaluate baseline vital signs.
Provide oxygen	Provide supplementary oxygen to hypoxemic (eg, oxyhemoglobin saturation less than 94%) stroke patients or those patients with unknown oxygen saturation.
Establish IV access and obtain blood samples	Establish IV access and obtain blood samples for baseline blood count, coagulation studies, and blood glucose. Do not let this delay obtaining a CT scan of the brain.

(continued)

(continued)

Step	Actions
Check glucose	Promptly treat hypoglycemia.
Perform neurologic assessment	Perform a neurologic screening assessment. Use the NIH Stroke Scale (NIHSS) or a similar tool.
Activate the stroke team	Activate the stroke team or arrange consultation with a stroke expert based on predetermined protocols.
Order CT brain scan	Order an emergent CT scan of the brain. Have it read promptly by a qualified physician.
Obtain 12-lead ECG	Obtain a 12-lead ECG, which may identify a recent or ongoing AMI or arrhythmias (eg, atrial fibrillation) as a cause of embolic stroke. A small percentage of patients with acute stroke or transient ischemic attack have coexisting myocardial ischemia or other abnormalities. There is general agreement to recommend cardiac monitoring during the first 24 hours of evaluation in patients with acute ischemic stroke to detect atrial fibrillation and potentially life-threatening arrhythmias.
	Life-threatening arrhythmias can follow or accompany stroke, particularly intracerebral hemorrhage. If the patient is hemodynamically stable, treatment of non–life-threatening arrhythmias (bradycardia, VT, and atrioventricular [AV] conduction blocks) may not be necessary.
	Do not delay the CT scan to obtain the ECG.

Immediate Neurologic Assessment by Stroke Team or Designee

Overview

The stroke team, neurovascular consultant, or emergency physician does the following:

- Reviews the patient's history, performs a general physical examination, and establishes time of symptom onset
- Performs a neurologic examination (eg, NIHSS)

The goal for neurologic assessment is within 25 minutes of the patient's arrival in the ED: "time is brain" (Step 4).

Establish Symptom Onset

Establishing the time of symptom onset may require interviewing out-of-hospital providers, witnesses, and family members to determine the time the patient was last known to be normal.

Neurologic Examination

Assess the patient's neurologic status by using one of the more advanced stroke scales. Following is an example:

National Institutes of Health Stroke Scale

The NIHSS uses 15 items to assess the responsive stroke patient. This is a validated measure of stroke severity based on a detailed neurologic examination. A detailed discussion is beyond the scope of the ACLS Provider Course.

CT Scan: Hemorrhage or No Hemorrhage

Introduction

A critical decision point in the assessment of the patient with acute stroke is the performance and interpretation of a noncontrast CT scan to differentiate ischemic from hemorrhagic stroke. Assessment also includes identifying other structural abnormalities that may be responsible for the patient's symptoms or that represent contraindication to fibrinolytic therapy. The initial noncontrast CT scan is the most important test for a patient with acute stroke.

- If a CT scan is not readily available, stabilize and promptly transfer the patient to a facility with this capability.
- Do not give aspirin, heparin, or rtPA until the CT scan has ruled out intracranial hemorrhage.

The CT scan should be completed within 25 minutes of the patient's arrival in the ED and should be read within 45 minutes from ED arrival: "time is brain" (Step 5).

Decision Point: Hemorrhage or No Hemorrhage

Additional imaging techniques such as CT perfusion, CT angiography, or magnetic resonance imaging scans of patients with suspected stroke should be promptly interpreted by a physician skilled in neuroimaging interpretation. Obtaining these studies should not delay initiation of IV rtPA in eligible patients. The presence of hemorrhage versus no hemorrhage determines the next steps in treatment (Figures 29A and B).

Yes, Hemorrhage Is Present

If hemorrhage is noted on the CT scan, the patient is not a candidate for fibrinolytics. Consult a neurologist or neurosurgeon. Consider transfer for appropriate care (Step 7).

No, Hemorrhage Is Not Present

If the CT scan shows no evidence of hemorrhage and no sign of other abnormality (eg, tumor, recent stroke), the patient may be a candidate for fibrinolytic therapy (Steps 6 and 8).

If hemorrhage is not present on the initial CT scan and the patient is not a candidate for fibrinolytics for other reasons, consider giving aspirin (Step 9) either rectally or orally after performing a swallowing screen (see below). Although aspirin is not a time-critical intervention, it is appropriate to administer aspirin in the ED if the patient is not a candidate for fibrinolysis. The patient must be able to safely swallow before aspirin is given orally. Otherwise, use the suppository form.

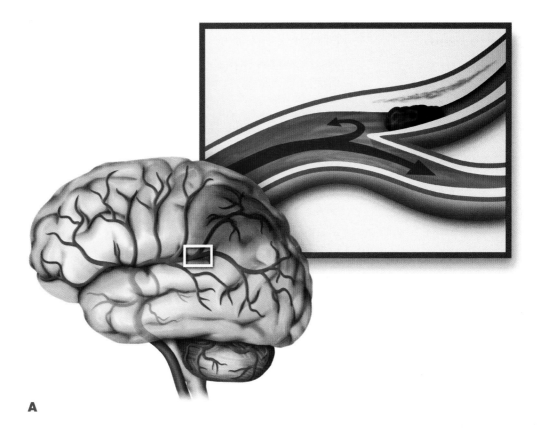

A

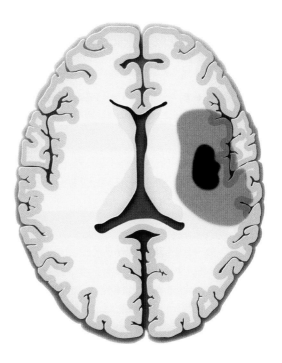

B

Figure 29. Occlusion in a cerebral artery by a thrombus. **A,** Area of infarction surrounding immediate site and distal portion of brain tissue after occlusion. **B,** Area of ischemic penumbra (ischemic, but not yet infarcted [dead] brain tissue) surrounding areas of infarction. This ischemic penumbra is alive but dysfunctional because of altered membrane potentials. The dysfunction is potentially reversible. Current stroke treatment tries to keep the area of permanent brain infarction as small as possible by preventing the areas of reversible brain ischemia in the penumbra from transforming into larger areas of irreversible brain infarction.

Fibrinolytic Therapy

Introduction

Several studies have shown a higher likelihood of good to excellent functional outcome when rtPA is given to adults with acute ischemic stroke within 3 hours of onset of symptoms, or within 4.5 hours of onset of symptoms for selected patients. But these results are obtained when rtPA is given by physicians in hospitals with a stroke protocol that rigorously adheres to the eligibility criteria and therapeutic regimen of the NINDS protocol. Evidence from prospective randomized studies in adults also documents a greater likelihood of benefit the earlier treatment begins.

The AHA and stroke guidelines recommend giving IV rtPA to patients with acute ischemic stroke who meet the NINDS eligibility criteria if it is given by

- Physicians using a clearly defined institutional protocol
- A knowledgeable interdisciplinary team familiar with stroke care
- An institution with a commitment to comprehensive stroke care and rehabilitation

The superior outcomes reported in both community and tertiary care hospitals in the NINDS trials can be difficult to replicate in hospitals with less experience in, and institutional commitment to, acute stroke care. There is strong evidence to avoid all delays and treat patients as soon as possible. Failure to adhere to protocol is associated with an increased rate of complications, particularly risk of intracranial hemorrhage.

Evaluate for Fibrinolytic Therapy

If the CT scan is negative for hemorrhage, the patient may be a candidate for fibrinolytic therapy. Immediately perform further eligibility and risk stratification:

- If the CT scan shows no hemorrhage, the probability of acute ischemic stroke remains. *Review inclusion and exclusion criteria for IV fibrinolytic therapy (Table 6) and repeat the neurologic exam* (NIHSS or Canadian Neurological Scale).
- If the patient's neurologic function is rapidly improving toward normal, fibrinolytics may be unnecessary.

Table 6. Inclusion and Exclusion Characteristics of Patients With Ischemic Stroke Who Could Be Treated With rtPA Within 3 Hours From Symptom Onset*

Inclusion Criteria
- Diagnosis of ischemic stroke causing measurable neurologic deficit
- Onset of symptoms <3 hours before beginning treatment
- Age ≥18 years

Exclusion Criteria
- Significant head trauma or prior stroke in previous 3 months
- Symptoms suggest subarachnoid hemorrhage
- Arterial puncture at noncompressible site in previous 7 days
- History of previous intracranial hemorrhage
– Intracranial neoplasm, arteriovenous malformation, or aneurysm
– Recent intracranial or intraspinal surgery
- Elevated blood pressure (systolic >185 mm Hg or diastolic >110 mm Hg)
- Active internal bleeding
- Acute bleeding diathesis, including but not limited to
– Platelet count <100 000/mm^3
– Heparin received within 48 hours, resulting in aPTT greater than the upper limit of normal
– Current use of anticoagulant with INR >1.7 or PT >15 seconds

(continued)

(continued)

> – Current use of direct thrombin inhibitors or direct factor Xa inhibitors with elevated sensitive laboratory tests (such as aPTT, INR, platelet count, and ECT; TT; or appropriate factor Xa activity assays)
> - Blood glucose concentration <50 mg/dL (2.7 mmol/L)
> - CT demonstrates multilobar infarction (hypodensity >⅓ cerebral hemisphere)

Relative Exclusion Criteria

Recent experience suggests that under some circumstances—with careful consideration and weighing of risk to benefit—patients may receive fibrinolytic therapy despite 1 or more relative contraindications. Consider risk to benefit of rtPA administration carefully if any one of these relative contraindications is present:

- Only minor or rapidly improving stroke symptoms (clearing spontaneously)
- Pregnancy
- Seizure at onset with postictal residual neurologic impairments
- Major surgery or serious trauma within previous 14 days
- Recent gastrointestinal or urinary tract hemorrhage (within previous 21 days)
- Recent acute myocardial infarction (within previous 3 months)

Notes

- The checklist includes some US FDA–approved indications and contraindications for administration of rtPA for acute ischemic stroke. Recent AHA/ASA guideline revisions may differ slightly from FDA criteria. A physician with expertise in acute stroke care may modify this list.
- Onset time is either witnessed or last known normal.
- In patients without recent use of oral anticoagulants or heparin, treatment with rtPA can be initiated before availability of coagulation study results but should be discontinued if INR is >1.7 or PT is elevated by local laboratory standards.
- In patients without history of thrombocytopenia, treatment with rtPA can be initiated before availability of platelet count but should be discontinued if platelet count is <100 000/mm³.

Abbreviations: aPTT, activated partial thromboplastin time; CT, computed tomography; ECT, ecarin clotting time; FDA, Food and Drug Administration; INR, international normalized ratio; PT, prothrombin time; rtPA, recombinant tissue plasminogen activator; TT, thrombin time.

*Jauch EC, Saver JL, Adams HP Jr, et al. Guidelines for the early management of patients with acute ischemic stroke: a guideline for healthcare professionals from the American Heart Association/American Stroke Association. *Stroke*. 2013;44(3):870-947.

Potential Adverse Effects

As with all drugs, fibrinolytics have potential adverse effects. At this point, weigh the patient's risk for adverse events against the potential benefit and discuss with the patient and family.

- Confirm that no exclusion criteria are present (Table 6).
- Consider risks and benefits.
- Be prepared to monitor and treat any potential complications.

The major complication of IV rtPA for stroke is intracranial hemorrhage. Other bleeding complications may occur and may range from minor to major. Angioedema and transient hypotension may occur.

Patient Is a Candidate for Fibrinolytic Therapy

If the patient remains a candidate for fibrinolytic therapy (Step 8), discuss the risks and potential benefits with the patient or family if available (Step 10). After this discussion, if the patient or family members decide to proceed with fibrinolytic therapy, give the patient rtPA. Begin your institution's stroke rtPA protocol, often called a "pathway of care."

Do not administer anticoagulants or antiplatelet treatment for 24 hours after administration of rtPA, typically until a follow-up CT scan at 24 hours shows no intracranial hemorrhage.

Extended IV rtPA Window 3 to 4.5 Hours

Treatment of carefully selected patients with acute ischemic stroke with IV rtPA between 3 and 4.5 hours after onset of symptoms has also been shown to improve clinical outcome, although the degree of clinical benefit is smaller than that achieved with treatment within 3 hours. Data supporting treatment in this time window come from a large, randomized trial (ECASS-3 [European Cooperative Acute Stroke Study]) that specifically enrolled patients between 3 and 4.5 hours after symptom onset, as well as a meta-analysis of prior trials.

At present, use of IV rtPA within the 3- to 4.5-hour window has not yet been approved by the US Food and Drug Administration (FDA), although it is recommended by an AHA/American Stroke Association science advisory. Administration of IV rtPA to patients with acute ischemic stroke who meet the NINDS or ECASS-3 eligibility criteria (Table 7) is recommended if rtPA is administered by physicians in the setting of a clearly defined protocol, a knowledgeable team, and institutional commitment.

Table 7. Additional Inclusion and Exclusion Characteristics of Patients With Acute Ischemic Stroke Who Could Be Treated With IV rtPA Within *3 to 4.5 Hours* From Symptom Onset*

Inclusion Criteria
• Diagnosis of ischemic stroke causing measurable neurologic deficit
• Onset of symptoms 3 to 4.5 hours before beginning treatment

Exclusion Criteria
• Age >80 years
• Severe stroke (NIHSS score >25)
• Taking an oral anticoagulant regardless of INR
• History of both diabetes and prior ischemic stroke

Abbreviations: INR, international normalized ratio; NIHSS, National Institutes of Health Stroke Scale; rtPA, recombinant tissue plasminogen activator.

*Del Zoppo GJ, Saver JL, Jauch EC, Adams HP Jr, American Heart Association Stroke Council. Expansion of the time window for treatment of acute ischemic stroke with intravenous tissue plasminogen activator: a science advisory from the American Heart Association/American Stroke Association. Stroke. 2009;40(8):2945-2948.

Intra-arterial rtPA

Improved outcome from use of cerebral intra-arterial rtPA has been documented. For patients with acute ischemic stroke who are not candidates for standard IV fibrinolysis, consider intra-arterial fibrinolysis in centers with the resources and expertise to provide it within the first 6 hours after onset of symptoms. Intra-arterial administration of rtPA is not yet approved by the FDA.

Change

Simply measuring and benchmarking care can positively influence outcome. However, ongoing review and interpretation are necessary to identify areas for improvement, such as

- Citizen awareness
- Citizen and healthcare professional education and training
- Increased bystander CPR response rates
- Improved CPR performance
- Shortened time to defibrillation

Rhythms for VF/ Pulseless VT

This case involves these ECG rhythms:

- VF (example in Figure 30)
- VT
- ECG artifact that looks like VF
- New LBBB

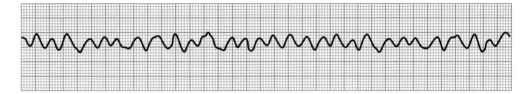

Figure 30. Example of ventricular fibrillation.

Drugs for VF/ Pulseless VT

This case involves these drugs:

- Epinephrine
- Norepinephrine
- Amiodarone
- Lidocaine
- Magnesium sulfate
- Dopamine
- Oxygen
- Other medications, depending on the cause of the VT/pulseless VT arrest

Managing VF/Pulseless VT: The Adult Cardiac Arrest Algorithm

Overview

The Adult Cardiac Arrest Algorithm (Figure 31) is the most important algorithm to know for adult resuscitation. This algorithm outlines all assessment and management steps for the pulseless patient who does not initially respond to BLS interventions, including a first shock from an AED. The algorithm consists of the 2 pathways for a cardiac arrest:

- A shockable rhythm (VF/pulseless VT) displayed on the left side of the algorithm
- A nonshockable rhythm (asystole/PEA) displayed on the right side of the algorithm

Throughout the case discussion of the Cardiac Arrest Algorithm, we will refer to Steps 1 through 12. These are the numbers assigned to the steps in the algorithm.

VF/pVT (Left Side)

Because many patients with sudden cardiac arrest demonstrate VF at some point in their arrest, it is likely that ACLS providers will frequently follow the left side of the Cardiac Arrest Algorithm (Figure 31). Rapid treatment of VF according to this sequence is the best approach to restoring spontaneous circulation.

Pulseless VT is included in the algorithm because it is treated as VF. VF and pulseless VT require CPR until a defibrillator is available. Both are treated with high-energy unsynchronized shocks.

Asystole/PEA (Right Side)

The right side of the algorithm outlines the sequence of actions to perform if the rhythm is nonshockable. You will have an opportunity to practice this sequence in the Asystole and PEA Cases.

Summary

The VF/Pulseless VT Case gives you the opportunity to practice performing rapid treatment of VF/pVT by following the steps on the left side of the Cardiac Arrest Algorithm (Steps 1 through 8).

Adult Cardiac Arrest Algorithm—2015 Update

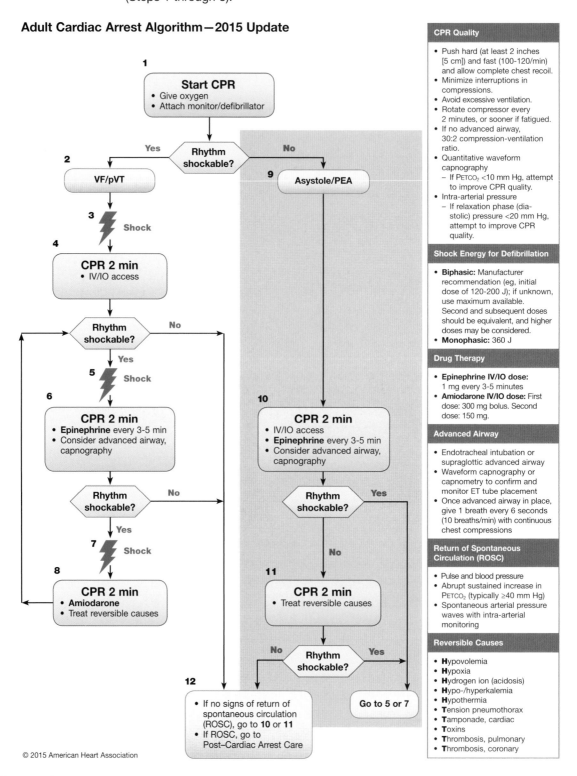

© 2015 American Heart Association

Figure 31. The Adult Cardiac Arrest Algorithm.

Application of the Adult Cardiac Arrest Algorithm: VF/pVT Pathway

Introduction

This case discusses the assessment and treatment of a patient with refractory VF or pulseless VT. This algorithm assumes that healthcare providers have completed the BLS Assessment, including activation of the emergency response system, performing CPR, attaching the manual defibrillator, and delivering the first shock (Steps 1 through 4).

The ACLS high-performance team now intervenes and conducts the Primary Assessment. In this case, the team assesses the patient and takes actions as needed. The team leader coordinates the efforts of the high-performance team as they perform the steps listed in the VF/pVT pathway on the left side of the Cardiac Arrest Algorithm.

Minimal Interruption of Chest Compressions

A team member should continue to perform high-quality CPR until the defibrillator arrives and is attached to the patient. The team leader assigns roles and responsibilities and organizes interventions to minimize interruptions in chest compressions. This accomplishes the most critical interventions for VF or pulseless VT: CPR with minimal interruptions in chest compressions and defibrillation during the first minutes of arrest.

The AHA does not recommend continued use of an AED (or the automatic mode) when a manual defibrillator is available and the provider's skills are adequate for rhythm interpretation. Rhythm analysis and shock administration with an AED may result in prolonged interruptions in chest compressions.

Figure 32 demonstrates the need to minimize interruptions in compressions. CPP is aortic relaxation ("diastolic") pressure minus right atrial relaxation ("diastolic") pressure. During CPR, CPP correlates with both myocardial blood flow and ROSC. In 1 human study, ROSC did not occur unless a CPP 15 mm Hg or greater was achieved during CPR.

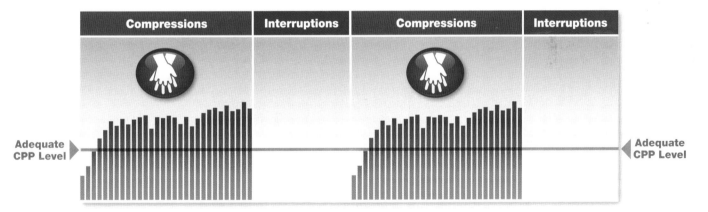

Figure 32. Relationship of quality CPR to coronary perfusion pressure (CPP) demonstrating the need to minimize interruptions in compressions.

Resume CPR While Manual Defibrillator Is Charging

- Shortening the interval between the last compression and the shock by even a few seconds can improve shock success (defibrillation and ROSC). Thus, it is reasonable for healthcare providers to practice efficient coordination between CPR and defibrillation to minimize the hands-off interval between stopping compressions and administering the shock.

- For example, after verifying a shockable rhythm and initiating the charging sequence on the defibrillator, another provider should resume chest compressions and continue until the defibrillator is fully charged. The defibrillator operator should deliver the shock as soon as the compressor removes his or her hands from the patient's chest and all providers are "clear" of contact with the patient.

- Use of a multimodal defibrillator in manual mode may reduce the duration of chest compression interruption required for rhythm analysis compared with automatic mode but could increase the frequency of inappropriate shock. Individuals who are not comfortable interpreting cardiac rhythms can continue to use an AED.

- For an AED, follow the device's prompts or know your device-specific manufacturer's recommendations.

- It is important that healthcare providers be knowledgeable of how their defibrillator operates, and if possible, limit pauses in chest compressions to rhythm analysis and shock delivery.

Deliver 1 Shock

Step 3 directs you to deliver 1 shock. The appropriate energy dose is determined by the identity of the defibrillator—monophasic or biphasic. See the column on the right of the algorithm.

If you are using a *monophasic* defibrillator, give a single 360-J shock. Use the same energy dose for subsequent shocks.

Biphasic defibrillators use a variety of waveforms, each of which is effective for terminating VF over a specific dose range. When using biphasic defibrillators, providers should use the manufacturer's recommended energy dose (eg, initial dose of 120 to 200 J). Many biphasic defibrillator manufacturers display the effective energy dose range on the face of the device. If you do not know the effective dose range, deliver the maximal energy dose for the first and all subsequent shocks.

If the initial shock terminates VF but the arrhythmia recurs later in the resuscitation attempt, deliver subsequent shocks at the previously successful energy level.

Immediately after the shock, resume CPR, beginning with chest compressions. Give 2 minutes of CPR.

Purpose of Defibrillation

Defibrillation does not restart the heart. Defibrillation stuns the heart and briefly terminates all electrical activity, including VF and pVT. If the heart is still viable, its normal pacemakers may eventually resume electrical activity (return of spontaneous rhythm) that ultimately results in a perfusing rhythm (ROSC).

In the first minutes after successful defibrillation, however, any spontaneous rhythm is typically slow and may not create pulses or adequate perfusion. The patient needs CPR (beginning with chest compressions) for several minutes until adequate heart function resumes. Moreover, not all shocks will lead to successful defibrillation. This is why it is important to resume high-quality CPR, beginning with chest compressions immediately after a shock.

Principle of Early Defibrillation

The interval from collapse to defibrillation is one of the most important determinants of survival from cardiac arrest. Early defibrillation is critical for patients with sudden cardiac arrest for the following reasons:

- A common initial rhythm in out-of-hospital witnessed sudden cardiac arrest is VF. Pulseless VT rapidly deteriorates to VF. When VF is present, the heart quivers and does not pump blood.
- Electrical defibrillation is the most effective way to treat VF (delivery of a shock to stop the VF).
- The probability of successful defibrillation decreases quickly over time.
- VF deteriorates to asystole if not treated.

The earlier defibrillation occurs, the higher the survival rate. When VF is present, CPR can provide a small amount of blood flow to the heart and brain but cannot directly restore an organized rhythm. The likelihood of restoring a perfusing rhythm is optimized with immediate CPR and defibrillation within a few minutes of the initial arrest (Figure 33).

For every minute that passes between collapse and defibrillation, the chance of survival from a witnessed VF sudden cardiac arrest declines by 7% to 10% per minute if no bystander CPR is provided.[3] When bystanders perform CPR, the decline is more gradual and averages 3% to 4% per minute.[3-6] CPR performed early can double[3,7] or triple[8] survival from witnessed sudden cardiac arrest at most defibrillation intervals.

Lay rescuer AED programs increase the likelihood of early CPR and attempted defibrillation. This helps shorten the time between collapse and defibrillation for a greater number of patients with sudden cardiac arrest.

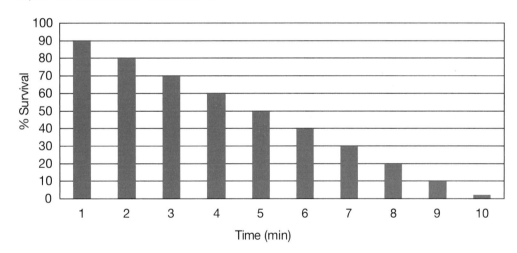

Figure 33. Relationship between survival from ventricular fibrillation sudden cardiac arrest and time from collapse to defibrillation.

Foundational Facts

Clearing for Defibrillation

To ensure safety during defibrillation, always announce the shock warning. State the warning firmly and in a forceful voice before delivering each shock (this entire sequence should take less than 5 seconds):

- **"Clear. Shocking."**
  - Check to make sure you are clear of contact with the patient, the stretcher, or other equipment.
  - Make a visual check to ensure that no one is touching the patient or stretcher.
  - Be sure oxygen is not flowing across the patient's chest.
- When pressing the shock button, the defibrillator operator should face the patient, not the machine. This helps to ensure coordination with the chest compressor and to verify that no one resumed contact with the patient.

You do not need to use these exact words, but you must warn others that you are about to deliver shocks and that everyone must stand clear of the patient.

Resume CPR

- Immediately resume CPR, beginning with chest compressions.
- Do not perform a rhythm or pulse check at this point unless the patient is showing signs of life or advanced monitoring indicates ROSC.
- Establish IV/IO access.

The Guidelines recommend that healthcare providers tailor the sequence of rescue actions based on the presumed etiology of the arrest. Moreover, ACLS providers functioning within a high-performance team can choose the optimal approach for minimizing interruptions in chest compressions (thereby improving chest compression fraction). Use of different protocols, such as 3 cycles of 200 continuous compressions with passive oxygen insufflation and airway adjuncts, compression-only CPR in the first few minutes after arrest, and continuous chest compressions with asynchronous ventilation once every 6 seconds with the use of a bag-mask device, are a few examples of optimizing CCF and high-quality CPR. A default compression-to-ventilation ratio of 30:2 should be used by less-trained healthcare providers or if 30:2 is the established protocol. Figure 34 shows the progression from lay rescuers to highly trained and proficient healthcare providers.

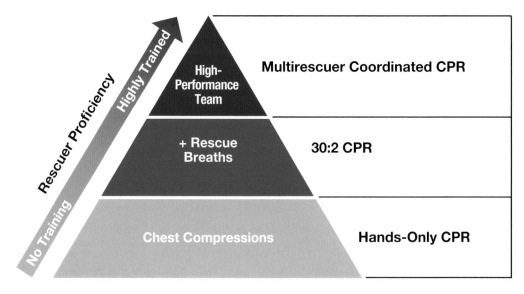

Figure 34. Progression from lay rescuers to highly trained healthcare providers for CPR delivery.

Rhythm Check

Conduct a rhythm check after 2 minutes of CPR. Be careful to minimize interruptions in chest compressions.

The pause in chest compressions to check the rhythm should not exceed 10 seconds.

- If a nonshockable rhythm is present and the rhythm is organized, a team member should try to palpate a pulse. If there is any doubt about the presence of a pulse, immediately resume CPR.

Remember: *Perform a pulse check—preferably during rhythm analysis—only if an organized rhythm is present.*

- If the rhythm is organized and there is a palpable pulse, proceed to post–cardiac arrest care.
- If the rhythm check reveals a nonshockable rhythm and there is no pulse, proceed along the asystole/PEA pathway on the right side of the Cardiac Arrest Algorithm (Steps 9 through 11).
- If the rhythm check reveals a shockable rhythm, give 1 shock and resume CPR immediately for 2 minutes after the shock (Step 6).

Self-Adhesive Pads

The AHA recommends routine use of self-adhesive pads. Using conductive materials (gel pads or self-adhesive pads) during the defibrillation attempt reduces transthoracic impedance, or the resistance that chest structures have on electrical current.

Shock and Vasopressors

For persistent VF/pulseless VT, give 1 shock and resume CPR immediately for 2 minutes after the shock.

Immediately after the shock, resume CPR, beginning with chest compressions. Give 2 minutes of CPR.

When IV/IO access is available, give epinephrine during CPR after the second shock as follows:

- **Epinephrine** 1 mg IV/IO—repeat every 3 to 5 minutes

Note: If additional team members are available, they should anticipate the need for drugs and prepare them in advance.

Epinephrine hydrochloride is used during resuscitation primarily for its β-adrenergic effects, ie, vasoconstriction. Vasoconstriction increases cerebral and coronary blood flow during CPR by increasing mean arterial pressure and aortic diastolic pressure. In previous studies, escalating and high-dose epinephrine administration did not improve survival to discharge or neurologic outcome after resuscitation from cardiac arrest.

No known vasopressor (epinephrine) increases survival from VF/pulseless VT. Because these medications can improve aortic diastolic blood pressure, coronary artery perfusion pressure, and the rate of ROSC, the AHA continues to recommend their use.

FYI 2015 Guidelines

Vasopressin

Vasopressin has been removed from the *2015 AHA Guidelines Update for CPR and ECC.*

The *2015 AHA Guidelines Update for CPR and ECC* states that "vasopressin offers no advantage as a substitute for epinephrine in cardiac arrest." As such, it has been removed from the 2015 updated Adult Cardiac Arrest Algorithm.

Rhythm Check

Conduct a rhythm check after 2 minutes of CPR. Be careful to minimize interruptions in chest compressions.

Interruption in compressions to conduct a rhythm analysis should not exceed 10 seconds.

- If a nonshockable rhythm is present and the rhythm is organized, a team member should try to palpate a pulse. If there is any doubt about the presence of a pulse, immediately resume CPR.
- If the rhythm check is organized and there is a palpable pulse, proceed to post–cardiac arrest care.
- If the rhythm check reveals a nonshockable rhythm and there is no pulse, proceed along the asystole/PEA pathway on the right side of the Cardiac Arrest Algorithm (Steps 9 through 11).
- If the rhythm check reveals a shockable rhythm, resume chest compressions if indicated while the defibrillator is charging (Step 8). The team leader is responsible for team safety while compressions are being performed and the defibrillator is charging.

Shock and Antiarrhythmics

Give 1 shock and resume CPR beginning with chest compressions for 2 minutes immediately after the shock.

Healthcare providers may consider giving antiarrhythmic drugs, either before or after the shock. Research is still lacking on the effect of antiarrhythmic drugs given during cardiac arrest on survival to hospital discharge. If administered, amiodarone is the first-line antiarrhythmic agent given in cardiac arrest because it has been clinically demonstrated that it improves the rate of ROSC and hospital admission in adults with refractory VF/pulseless VT.

- **Amiodarone** 300 mg IV/IO bolus, then consider an additional 150 mg IV/IO once
  - Amiodarone is considered a class III antiarrhythmic drug, but it possesses electrophysiologic characteristics of the other classes. Amiodarone blocks sodium channels at rapid pacing frequencies (class I effect) and exerts a noncompetitive antisympathetic action (class II effect). One of the main effects of prolonged amiodarone administration is lengthening of the cardiac action potential (class III effect).

If amiodarone is not available, providers may administer lidocaine.

- **Lidocaine** 1 to 1.5 mg/kg IV/IO first dose, then 0.5 to 0.75 mg/kg IV/IO at 5- to 10-minute intervals, to a maximum dose of 3 mg/kg
  - Lidocaine suppresses automaticity of conduction tissue in the heart, by increasing the electrical stimulation threshold of the ventricle, His-Purkinje system, and spontaneous depolarization of the ventricles during diastole by a direct action on the tissues.
  - Lidocaine blocks permeability of the neuronal membrane to sodium ions, which results in inhibition of depolarization and the blockade of conduction.

Providers should consider magnesium sulfate for torsades de pointes associated with a long QT interval.

- **Magnesium sulfate** for torsades de pointes, loading dose 1 to 2 g IV/IO diluted in 10 mL (eg, D_5W, normal saline) given as IV/IO bolus, typically over 5 to 20 minutes
  - Magnesium can be classified as a sodium/potassium pump agonist.
  - Magnesium has several electrophysiological effects, including suppression of atrial L- and T-type calcium channels, and ventricular after-depolarizations.

Routine administration of magnesium sulfate in cardiac arrest is not recommended unless torsades de pointes is present.

Search for and treat any treatable underlying cause of cardiac arrest. See the column on the right of the algorithm. See Table 4 in Part 4 for more information on the H's and T's.

Cardiac Arrest Treatment Sequences

The Adult Cardiac Arrest Circular Algorithm (Figure 35) summarizes the recommended sequence of CPR, rhythm checks, shocks, and delivery of drugs based on expert consensus. The optimal number of cycles of CPR and shocks required before starting pharmacologic therapy remains unknown. Note that rhythm checks and shocks are organized around 5 cycles of compressions and ventilations, or 2 minutes if a provider is timing the arrest.

Adult Cardiac Arrest Circular Algorithm—2015 Update

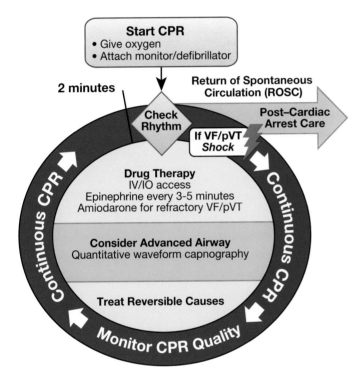

© 2015 American Heart Association

CPR Quality

- Push hard (at least 2 inches [5 cm]) and fast (100-120/min) and allow complete chest recoil.
- Minimize interruptions in compressions.
- Avoid excessive ventilation.
- Rotate compressor every 2 minutes, or sooner if fatigued.
- If no advanced airway, 30:2 compression-ventilation ratio.
- Quantitative waveform capnography
  - If P_{ETCO_2} <10 mm Hg, attempt to improve CPR quality.
- Intra-arterial pressure
  - If relaxation phase (diastolic) pressure <20 mm Hg, attempt to improve CPR quality.

Shock Energy for Defibrillation

- **Biphasic:** Manufacturer recommendation (eg, initial dose of 120-200 J); if unknown, use maximum available. Second and subsequent doses should be equivalent, and higher doses may be considered.
- **Monophasic:** 360 J

Drug Therapy

- **Epinephrine IV/IO dose:** 1 mg every 3-5 minutes
- **Amiodarone IV/IO dose:** First dose: 300 mg bolus. Second dose: 150 mg.

Advanced Airway

- Endotracheal intubation or supraglottic advanced airway
- Waveform capnography or capnometry to confirm and monitor ET tube placement
- Once advanced airway in place, give 1 breath every 6 seconds (10 breaths/min) with continuous chest compressions

Return of Spontaneous Circulation (ROSC)

- Pulse and blood pressure
- Abrupt sustained increase in P_{ETCO_2} (typically ≥40 mm Hg)
- Spontaneous arterial pressure waves with intra-arterial monitoring

Reversible Causes

- **H**ypovolemia
- **H**ypoxia
- **H**ydrogen ion (acidosis)
- **H**ypo-/hyperkalemia
- **H**ypothermia

- **T**ension pneumothorax
- **T**amponade, cardiac
- **T**oxins
- **T**hrombosis, pulmonary
- **T**hrombosis, coronary

Figure 35. The Adult Cardiac Arrest Circular Algorithm. Do not delay shock. Continue CPR while preparing and administering drugs and charging the defibrillator. Interrupt chest compressions only for the minimum amount of time required for ventilation (until advanced airway placed), rhythm check, and actual shock delivery.

Physiologic Monitoring During CPR

The AHA recommends using quantitative waveform capnography in intubated patients to monitor CPR quality (Figure 36), optimize chest compressions, and detect ROSC during chest compressions (Figure 37). Although placement of invasive monitors during CPR is not generally warranted, physiologic parameters such as intra-arterial relaxation pressures (Figures 36A and B) and central venous oxygen saturation ($SCVO_2$), when available, may also be helpful for optimizing CPR and detecting ROSC.

Animal and human studies indicate that $PETCO_2$, CPP, and $SCVO_2$ monitoring provides valuable information on both the patient's condition and the response to therapy. Most important, $PETCO_2$, CPP, and $SCVO_2$ correlate with cardiac output and myocardial blood flow during CPR. When chest compressions fail to achieve identified threshold values, ROSC is rarely achieved. Furthermore, an abrupt increase in any of these parameters is a sensitive indicator of ROSC that can be monitored without interrupting chest compressions.

Although no clinical study has examined whether titrating resuscitative efforts to physiologic parameters improves outcome, it is reasonable to use these parameters, if available, to optimize compressions and guide vasopressor therapy during cardiac arrest.

End-Tidal CO_2

The main determinant of $PETCO_2$ during CPR is blood delivery to the lungs. Persistently low $PETCO_2$ values less than 10 mm Hg during CPR in intubated patients (Figure 36B) suggest that ROSC is unlikely. If $PETCO_2$ abruptly increases to a normal value of 35 to 40 mm Hg, it is reasonable to consider this an indicator of ROSC.

- If the $PETCO_2$ is less than 10 mm Hg during CPR, it is reasonable to try to improve chest compressions and vasopressor therapy.

Coronary Perfusion Pressure or Arterial Relaxation Pressure

Increased CPP correlates with both myocardial blood flow and ROSC. A reasonable surrogate for CPP during CPR is arterial relaxation ("diastolic") pressure, which can be measured by using an intra-arterial catheter.

- If the arterial relaxation pressure is less than 20 mm Hg (Figure 36B), it is reasonable to try to improve chest compressions and vasopressor therapy.

Central Venous Oxygen Saturation

If oxygen consumption, arterial oxygen saturation, and hemoglobin are constant, changes in $SCVO_2$ reflect changes in oxygen delivery due to changes in cardiac output. $SCVO_2$ can be measured continuously by using oximetric tipped central venous catheters placed in the superior vena cava or pulmonary artery. Normal range is 60% to 80%.

- If the $SCVO_2$ is less than 30%, it is reasonable to try to improve chest compressions and vasopressor therapy.

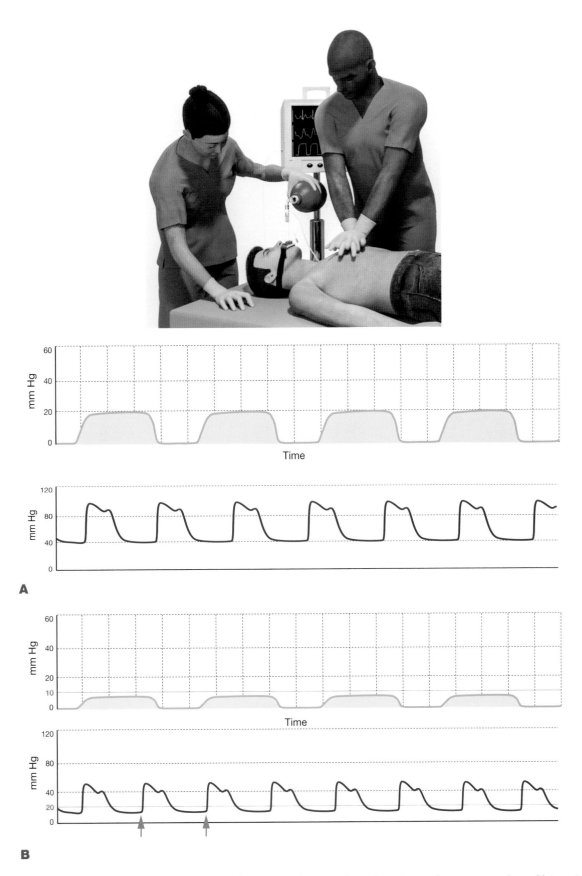

Figure 36. Physiologic monitoring during CPR. **A,** High-quality compressions are shown through waveform capnography and intra-arterial relaxation pressure. PETCO₂ values less than 10 mm Hg in intubated patients or intra-arterial relaxation pressures less than 20 mm Hg indicate that cardiac output is inadequate to achieve ROSC. In either of those cases, it is reasonable to consider trying to improve quality of CPR by optimizing chest compression parameters or giving a vasopressor or both. **B,** Ineffective CPR compressions shown through intra-arterial relaxation pressure and waveform capnography.

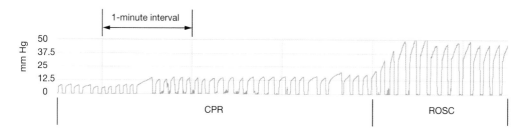

Figure 37. Waveform capnography during CPR with ROSC. This capnography tracing displays PETCO₂ in millimeters of mercury on the vertical axis over time. This patient is intubated and receiving CPR. Note that the ventilation rate is approximately 10/min. Chest compressions are given continuously at a rate slightly faster than 100/min but are not visible with this tracing. The initial PETCO₂ is less than 12.5 mm Hg during the first minute, indicating very low blood flow. PETCO₂ increases to between 12.5 and 25 mm Hg during the second and third minutes, consistent with the increase in blood flow with ongoing resuscitation. ROSC occurs during the fourth minute. ROSC is recognized by the abrupt increase in PETCO₂ (visible just after the fourth vertical line) to greater than 50 mm Hg, which is consistent with a substantial improvement in blood flow.

Treatment of VF/pVT in Hypothermia

Defibrillation is appropriate for the cardiac arrest patient in VF/pVT who has severe hypothermia and a body temperature of less than 30°C (less than 86°F). If the patient does not respond to the initial shock, it is reasonable to perform additional defibrillation attempts according to the usual BLS guidelines while engaging in active rewarming. The hypothermic patient may have a reduced rate of drug metabolism, raising concern that drug levels may accumulate to toxic levels with standard dosing regimens. Although the evidence does not support the use of antiarrhythmic drug therapy in hypothermic patients in cardiac arrest, it is reasonable to consider administration of a vasopressor according to the standard ACLS algorithm concurrent with rewarming strategies.

ACLS treatment of the patient with severe hypothermia in cardiac arrest in the hospital should be aimed at rapid core rewarming.

For patients in cardiac arrest with moderate hypothermia (30°C to 34°C [86°F to 93.2°F]), start CPR, attempt defibrillation, give medications spaced at longer intervals, and, if in hospital, provide active core rewarming.

Routes of Access for Drugs

Priorities

Priorities during cardiac arrest are high-quality CPR and early defibrillation. Insertion of an advanced airway and drug administration are of secondary importance. No drug given during cardiac arrest has been studied adequately to show improved survival to hospital discharge or improved neurologic function after cardiac arrest.

Historically in ACLS, providers have administered drugs either via the IV or ET route. ET absorption of drugs is poor and optimal drug dosing is not known. For this reason, the IV or IO route is preferred.

Intravenous Route

A peripheral IV is preferred for drug and fluid administration unless central line access is already available.

Central line access is not necessary during most resuscitation attempts. Central line access may cause interruptions in CPR and complications during insertion, including vascular laceration, hematomas, and bleeding. Insertion of a central line in a noncompressible vessel is a relative (not absolute) contraindication to fibrinolytic therapy in patients with ACS.

Extracorporeal CPR (for VF/Pulseless VT/Asystole/PEA)

Extracorporeal Membrane Oxygenation

Extracorporeal CPR (ECPR) refers to venoarterial extracorporeal membrane oxygenation during cardiac arrest, including extracorporeal membrane oxygenation and cardiopulmonary bypass. These techniques require adequate vascular access and specialized equipment. The use of ECPR may allow providers additional time to treat reversible underlying causes of cardiac arrest (eg, acute coronary artery occlusion, PE, refractory VF, profound hypothermia, cardiac injury, myocarditis, cardiomyopathy, congestive heart failure, drug intoxication) or serve as a bridge for LV assist device implantation or cardiac transplantation.

While there are currently no data from RCTs on the use of ECPR for cardiac arrest, evidence reviewed for the *2015 AHA Guidelines Update for CPR and ECC* suggests a benefit to survival and favorable neurologic outcome with the use of ECPR when compared with conventional CPR in patients with refractory cardiac arrest.

In settings where ECPR can be rapidly implemented, providers may consider its use among select cardiac arrest patients with potentially reversible causes of cardiac arrest who have not responded to initial conventional CPR.

Ultrasound (for VF/Pulseless VT/Asystole/PEA)

Ultrasound Use in Cardiac Arrest

Ultrasound may be applied to patients receiving CPR to help assess myocardial contractility and to help identify potentially treatable causes of cardiac arrest, such as hypovolemia, pneumothorax, pulmonary thromboembolism, or pericardial tamponade. However, it is unclear whether important clinical outcomes are affected by the routine use of ultrasound among patients experiencing cardiac arrest. If a qualified sonographer is present and use of ultrasound does not interfere with the standard cardiac arrest treatment protocol, then ultrasound may be considered as an adjunct to standard patient evaluation.

Cardiac Arrest: Pulseless Electrical Activity Case

Introduction	This case focuses on assessment and management of a *cardiac arrest patient with PEA*. During the BLS Assessment, high-performance team members will demonstrate high-quality CPR with effective chest compressions and ventilation with a bag-mask device. In the Primary Assessment, the team leader will recognize PEA and implement the appropriate interventions outlined in the Cardiac Arrest Algorithm. Because correction of an underlying cause of PEA, if present and identified, is critical to patient outcome, the team leader will verbalize the differential diagnosis while leading the high-performance team in the search for and treatment of reversible causes.
Rhythms for PEA	You will need to recognize the following rhythms: <ul><li>Rate—too fast or too slow</li><li>Width of QRS complexes—wide versus narrow</li></ul>
Drugs for PEA	This case involves these drugs: <ul><li>Epinephrine</li><li>Other medications, depending on the cause of the PEA arrest</li></ul>

Description of PEA

Introduction	PEA encompasses a heterogeneous group of rhythms that are organized or semiorganized but lack a palpable pulse. PEA includes <ul><li>Idioventricular rhythms</li><li>Ventricular escape rhythms</li><li>Postdefibrillation idioventricular rhythms</li><li>Sinus rhythm</li><li>Other</li></ul> Any organized* rhythm without a pulse is defined as PEA. Even sinus rhythm without a detectable pulse is called PEA. Pulseless rhythms that are excluded by definition include VF, pVT, and asystole. *An organized rhythm consists of QRS complexes that are similar in appearance from beat to beat (ie, each has a uniform QRS configuration). Organized rhythms may have narrow or wide QRS complexes, they may occur at rapid or slow rates, they may be regular or irregular, and they may or may not produce a pulse.
Historical Perspective	Previously, high-performance teams used the term *electromechanical dissociation* (EMD) to describe patients who displayed electrical activity on the cardiac monitor but lacked apparent contractile function because of an undetectable pulse. That is, weak contractile function is present—detectable by invasive monitoring or echocardiography—but the cardiac function is too weak to produce a pulse or effective cardiac output. This is the most common initial condition present after successful defibrillation. PEA also includes other conditions where the heart is empty because of inadequate preload. In this case, the contractile function of the heart is adequate, but there is inadequate volume for the ventricle to eject. This may occur as a result of severe hypovolemia, or as a result of decreased venous return from PE or pneumothorax.

Managing PEA: The Adult Cardiac Arrest Algorithm

Overview

As described earlier, the Cardiac Arrest Algorithm consists of 2 cardiac arrest pathways (Figure 39). The left side of the algorithm outlines treatment for a shockable rhythm (VF/pVT). The right side of the algorithm (Steps 9 through 11) outlines treatment for a non-shockable rhythm (asystole/PEA). Because of the similarity in causes and management, the Cardiac Arrest Algorithm combines the asystole and PEA pathways, although we will review these rhythms in separate cases. In both pathways, therapies are organized around periods (2 minutes) of uninterrupted, high-quality CPR.

The ability to achieve a good resuscitation outcome with return of a perfusing rhythm and spontaneous respirations depends on the ability of the high-performance team to provide effective CPR and to identify and correct a cause of PEA if present.

Everyone on the high-performance team must carry out the steps outlined in the algorithm and at the same time focus on the identification and treatment of reversible causes of the arrest.

The PEA Pathway of the Cardiac Arrest Algorithm

In this case, the *patient is in cardiac arrest.* High-performance team members initiate and perform high-quality CPR throughout the BLS Assessment and the Primary and Secondary Assessments. The team interrupts CPR for 10 seconds or less for rhythm and pulse checks. *This patient has an organized rhythm on the monitor but no pulse. The condition is PEA* (Step 9). Chest compressions resume immediately. The team leader now directs the team in the steps outlined in the PEA pathway of the Cardiac Arrest Algorithm (Figure 39), beginning with Step 10.

IV/IO access is a priority over advanced airway management unless bag-mask ventilation is ineffective or the arrest is caused by hypoxia. All high-performance team members must simultaneously conduct a search for an underlying and treatable cause of the PEA in addition to performing their assigned roles.

Decision Point: Rhythm Check

Conduct a rhythm check and give 2 minutes of CPR after administration of the drugs. Be careful to minimize interruptions in chest compressions.

The pause in CPR to conduct a rhythm check should not exceed 10 seconds.

Administer Epinephrine

- Give epinephrine as soon as IV/IO access becomes available.
  - Epinephrine 1 mg IV/IO—repeat every 3 to 5 minutes

Administer drugs during CPR. Do not stop CPR to administer drugs.

- Consider advanced airway and capnography.

Nonshockable Rhythm

- If *no electrical activity is present* (asystole), go back to Step 10.
- If organized electrical activity is present, try to palpate a pulse. Take at least 5 seconds but do not take more than 10 seconds to check for a pulse.
- If *no pulse is present*, or if there is any doubt about the presence of a pulse, immediately resume CPR for 2 minutes, starting with chest compressions. Go back to Step 10 and repeat the sequence.
- If a palpable pulse is present and the rhythm is organized, begin post–cardiac arrest care.

Adult Cardiac Arrest Algorithm—2015 Update

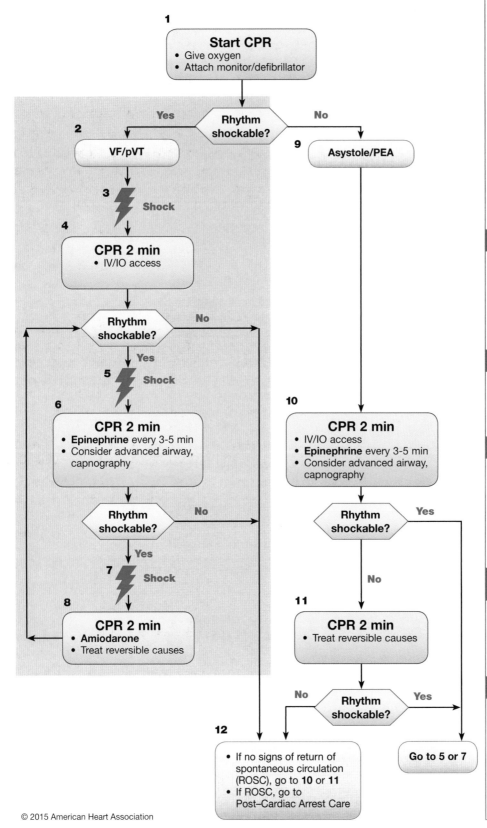

CPR Quality

- Push hard (at least 2 inches [5 cm]) and fast (100-120/min) and allow complete chest recoil.
- Minimize interruptions in compressions.
- Avoid excessive ventilation.
- Rotate compressor every 2 minutes, or sooner if fatigued.
- If no advanced airway, 30:2 compression-ventilation ratio.
- Quantitative waveform capnography
  – If P_{ETCO_2} <10 mm Hg, attempt to improve CPR quality.
- Intra-arterial pressure
  – If relaxation phase (diastolic) pressure <20 mm Hg, attempt to improve CPR quality.

Shock Energy for Defibrillation

- **Biphasic:** Manufacturer recommendation (eg, initial dose of 120-200 J); if unknown, use maximum available. Second and subsequent doses should be equivalent, and higher doses may be considered.
- **Monophasic:** 360 J

Drug Therapy

- **Epinephrine IV/IO dose:** 1 mg every 3-5 minutes
- **Amiodarone IV/IO dose:** First dose: 300 mg bolus. Second dose: 150 mg.

Advanced Airway

- Endotracheal intubation or supraglottic advanced airway
- Waveform capnography or capnometry to confirm and monitor ET tube placement
- Once advanced airway in place, give 1 breath every 6 seconds (10 breaths/min) with continuous chest compressions

Return of Spontaneous Circulation (ROSC)

- Pulse and blood pressure
- Abrupt sustained increase in P_{ETCO_2} (typically ≥40 mm Hg)
- Spontaneous arterial pressure waves with intra-arterial monitoring

Reversible Causes

- **H**ypovolemia
- **H**ypoxia
- **H**ydrogen ion (acidosis)
- **H**ypo-/hyperkalemia
- **H**ypothermia
- **T**ension pneumothorax
- **T**amponade, cardiac
- **T**oxins
- **T**hrombosis, pulmonary
- **T**hrombosis, coronary

Figure 39. The Adult Cardiac Arrest Algorithm.

Decision Point: Shockable Rhythm	• If the rhythm check reveals a shockable rhythm, resume CPR with chest compressions while the defibrillator is charging if possible.
	• Switch to the left side of the algorithm and perform steps according to the VF/pVT sequence starting with Step 5 or 7.

Asystole and PEA Treatment Sequences	Figure 39 summarizes the recommended sequence of CPR, rhythm checks, and delivery of drugs for PEA and asystole based on expert consensus.

Identification and Correction of Underlying Cause	Treatment of PEA is not limited to the interventions outlined in the algorithm. Healthcare providers should attempt to identify and correct an underlying cause if present. Healthcare providers must stop, think, and ask, "Why did this person have this cardiac arrest at this time?" It is essential to search for and treat reversible causes of asystole for resuscitative efforts to be potentially successful. Use the H's and T's to recall conditions that could have contributed to PEA.

Critical Concepts	**Common Underlying Causes of PEA**
	Hypovolemia and hypoxia are the 2 most common underlying and potentially reversible causes of PEA. Be sure to look for evidence of these problems as you assess the patient.

Cardiac Arrest: Asystole Case

Introduction	In this case, the *patient is in cardiac arrest.* High-performance team members initiate and perform high-quality CPR throughout the BLS Assessment and the Primary and Secondary Assessments. The team interrupts CPR for 10 seconds or less for a rhythm check. *This patient has no pulse and the rhythm on the monitor is asystole.* Chest compressions resume immediately. The team leader now directs the team in the steps outlined in the asystole pathway of the Cardiac Arrest Algorithm (Figure 31 in the section Managing VF/Pulseless VT: The Adult Cardiac Arrest Algorithm), beginning with Step 10.
	IV/IO access is a priority over advanced airway management unless bag-mask ventilation is ineffective or the arrest is caused by hypoxia. All high-performance team members must simultaneously conduct a search for an underlying and treatable cause of the asystole in addition to performing their assigned roles.
	At the end of this case, the team will discuss the criteria for terminating resuscitative efforts; in some cases, we must recognize that the patient is dead and that it would be more appropriate to direct efforts to supporting the family.

Rhythms for Asystole	You will need to recognize the following rhythms:
	• Asystole (example in Figure 40)
	• Slow PEA terminating in bradyasystolic rhythm

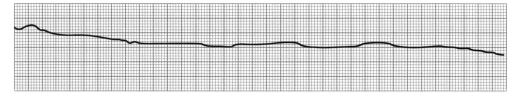

Figure 40. Example of asystole.

Drugs for Asystole	This case involves these drugs:
	• Epinephrine
	• Other medications, depending on the cause of the asystole arrest

Approach to Asystole

Introduction	Asystole is a cardiac arrest rhythm associated with no discernible electrical activity on the ECG (also referred to as *flat line*). You should confirm that the flat line on the monitor is indeed "true asystole" by validating that the flat line is
	• Not another rhythm (eg, fine VF) masquerading as a flat line
	• Not the result of an operator error

Foundational Facts	## Asystole and Technical Problems

Asystole is a specific diagnosis, but flat line is not. The term *flat line* is nonspecific and can result from several possible conditions, including absence of cardiac electrical activity, lead or other equipment failure, and operator error. Some defibrillators and monitors signal the operator when a lead or other equipment failure occurs. Some of these problems are not applicable to all defibrillators.

For a patient with cardiac arrest and asystole, quickly rule out any other causes of an isoelectric ECG, such as

- Loose leads or leads not connected to the patient or defibrillator/monitor
- No power
- Signal gain (amplitude/signal strength) too low

Patients With DNAR Orders

During the BLS, Primary, and Secondary Assessments, you should be aware of reasons to stop or withhold resuscitative efforts. Some of these are

- Rigor mortis
- Indicators of do-not-attempt-resuscitation (DNAR) status (eg, bracelet, anklet, written documentation)
- Threat to safety of providers

Out-of-hospital providers need to be aware of EMS-specific policies and protocols applicable to these situations. In-hospital providers and high-performance teams should be aware of advance directives or specific limits to resuscitation attempts that are in place. That is, some patients may consent to CPR and defibrillation but not to intubation or invasive procedures. Many hospitals will record this in the medical record.

Asystole as an End Point

Often, asystole represents the final rhythm. Cardiac function has diminished until electrical and functional cardiac activity finally stop and the patient dies. Asystole is also the final rhythm of a patient initially in VF or pVT.

Prolonged efforts are unnecessary and futile unless special resuscitation situations exist, such as hypothermia and drug overdose. Consider stopping if $ETCO_2$ is less than 10 after 20 minutes of CPR.

Managing Asystole

Overview

The management of asystole consists of the following components:

- Implementing the steps in the Cardiac Arrest Algorithm
- Identifying and correcting underlying causes
- Terminating efforts as appropriate

Adult Cardiac Arrest Algorithm

As described in the VF/Pulseless VT and PEA Cases, the Cardiac Arrest Algorithm consists of 2 pathways (Figures 31 and 39). The left side of the algorithm outlines treatment for a shockable rhythm (VF/pulseless VT). The right side of the algorithm (Steps 9 through 11) outlines treatment for a nonshockable rhythm (asystole/PEA). In both pathways, therapies are designed around periods (2 minutes) of uninterrupted, high-quality CPR. In this case, we will focus on the asystole component of the asystole/PEA pathway.

Identification and Correction of Underlying Cause

Treatment of asystole is not limited to the interventions outlined in the algorithm. Healthcare providers should attempt to identify and correct an underlying cause if present. Healthcare providers must stop, think, and ask, "Why did this person have this cardiac arrest at this time?" It is essential to search for and treat reversible causes of asystole for resuscitative efforts to be potentially successful. Use the H's and T's to recall conditions that could have contributed to asystole.

Application of the Adult Cardiac Arrest Algorithm: Asystole Pathway

Introduction

In this case, you have a patient in cardiac arrest. High-quality CPR is performed throughout the BLS, Primary, and Secondary Assessments. Interrupt CPR for 10 seconds or less while you perform a rhythm check. You interpret the rhythm on the monitor as asystole. CPR beginning with chest compressions for 2 minutes resumes immediately. You now conduct the steps outlined in the asystole pathway of the Cardiac Arrest Algorithm beginning with Step 9. At the same time, you are searching for a possible underlying cause of the asystole.

Confirmed Asystole

Give priority to IV/IO access. Do not interrupt CPR while establishing IV or IO access.

Administer Epinephrine

- Continue high-quality CPR, and as soon as IV/IO access is available, give epinephrine as follows:
  - **Epinephrine** 1 mg IV/IO—repeat every 3 to 5 minutes

Administer drugs during CPR. Do not stop CPR to administer drugs.

- Consider advanced airway and capnography.

Decision Point: Rhythm Check

Check the rhythm after 2 minutes of CPR.

Interruption of chest compressions to conduct a rhythm check should not exceed 10 seconds.

Nonshockable Rhythm

- If *no electrical activity is present* (asystole), go back to Step 10 or 11.
- If electrical activity is present and organized, try to palpate a pulse.
- If *no pulse is present* or if there is any doubt about the presence of a pulse, continue CPR, starting with chest compressions for 2 minutes. Go back to Step 10 and repeat the sequence.
- If a *good pulse is present and the rhythm is organized,* begin post–cardiac arrest care.

Shockable Rhythm

If the rhythm check reveals a shockable rhythm, prepare to deliver a shock (resuming chest compressions during charging if appropriate). Refer to the left side of the algorithm and perform steps according to the VF/pVT sequence, starting with Step 5 or 7.

Asystole and PEA Treatment Sequences

The diagram in Figure 39 (the Cardiac Arrest Algorithm) summarizes the recommended sequence of CPR, rhythm checks, and delivery of drugs for PEA and asystole based on expert consensus.

TCP Not Recommended

Several randomized controlled trials failed to show benefit from attempted TCP for asystole. The AHA does not recommend the use of TCP for patients with asystolic cardiac arrest.

Routine Shock Administration Not Recommended

There is no evidence that attempting to "defibrillate" asystole is beneficial. In one study, the group that received shocks had a trend toward worse outcome. Given the importance of minimizing interruption of chest compressions, there is no justification for interrupting chest compressions to deliver a shock to patients with asystole.

When in Doubt

If it is unclear whether the rhythm is fine VF or asystole, an initial attempt at defibrillation may be warranted. Fine VF may be the result of a prolonged arrest. At this time, the benefit of delaying defibrillation to perform CPR before defibrillation is unclear. EMS system medical directors may consider implementing a protocol that allows EMS responders to provide CPR while preparing for defibrillation of patients found by EMS personnel to be in VF.

Terminating Resuscitative Efforts

Terminating In-Hospital Resuscitative Efforts

If healthcare providers cannot rapidly identify an underlying cause and the patient does not respond to the BLS and ACLS interventions, termination of all resuscitative efforts should be considered.

The decision to terminate resuscitative efforts rests with the treating physician in the hospital and is based on consideration of many factors, including

- Time from collapse to CPR
- Time from collapse to first defibrillation attempt
- Comorbid disease
- Prearrest state
- Initial arrest rhythm
- Response to resuscitative measures
- $ETCO_2$ *less than 10 after 20 minutes of CPR*

None of these factors alone or in combination is clearly predictive of outcome. However, the duration of resuscitative efforts is an important factor associated with poor outcome. The chance that the patient will survive to hospital discharge and be neurologically intact diminishes as resuscitation time increases. Stop the resuscitation attempt when you determine with a high degree of certainty that the patient will not respond to further ACLS and ECPR is not indicated or not available.

Terminating Out-of-Hospital Resuscitative Efforts

Continue out-of-hospital resuscitative efforts until one of the following occurs:

- Restoration of effective, spontaneous circulation and ventilation
- Transfer of care to a senior emergency medical professional
- The presence of reliable criteria indicating irreversible death
- The healthcare provider is unable to continue because of exhaustion or dangerous environmental hazards or because continued resuscitation places the lives of others in jeopardy
- A valid DNAR order is presented
- Online authorization from the medical control physician or by prior medical protocol for termination of resuscitation

Duration of Resuscitative Efforts

The final decision to stop resuscitative efforts can never be as simple as an isolated time interval. If ROSC of any duration occurs, it may be appropriate to consider extending the resuscitative effort.

Experts have developed clinical rules to assist in decisions to terminate resuscitative efforts for in-hospital and out-of-hospital arrests. You should familiarize yourself with the established policy or protocols for your hospital or EMS system.

Continue out-of-hospital resuscitative efforts until one of the following occurs:

- Restoration of effective, spontaneous circulation and ventilation
- Transfer of care to a senior emergency medical professional
- The presence of reliable criteria indicating irreversible death
- The rescuer is unable to continue because of exhaustion or dangerous environmental hazards or because continued resuscitation places the lives of others in jeopardy
- A valid DNAR order is presented
- Online authorization from the medical control physician or by prior medical protocol for termination of resuscitation

It may also be appropriate to consider other issues, such as drug overdose and severe prearrest hypothermia (eg, submersion in icy water) when deciding whether to extend resuscitative efforts. Special resuscitation interventions and prolonged resuscitative efforts may be indicated for patients with hypothermia, drug overdose, or other potentially reversible causes of arrest.

Asystole: An Agonal Rhythm?

You will see asystole most frequently in 2 situations:

- As a terminal rhythm in a resuscitation attempt that started with another rhythm
- As the first rhythm identified in a patient with unwitnessed or prolonged arrest

Persistent asystole represents extensive myocardial ischemia and damage from prolonged periods of inadequate coronary perfusion. Prognosis is poor unless a special resuscitation circumstance or immediately reversible cause is present. Survival from asystole is better for in-hospital than for out-of-hospital arrests according to data from Get With The Guidelines®-Resuscitation, formerly the National Registry of CPR (**www.heart.org/resuscitation**).

Ethical Considerations

The high-performance team must make a conscientious and competent effort to give patients "a trial of CPR and ACLS," provided the patient had not expressed a decision to forego resuscitative efforts and the victim is not obviously dead (eg, rigor mortis, decomposition, hemisection, decapitation) (see the DNAR discussion on the Student Website). The final decision to stop resuscitative efforts can never be as simple as an isolated time interval.

 See Human, Ethical, and Legal Dimensions of CPR on the Student Website (**www.heart.org/eccstudent**).

Transport of Patients in Cardiac Arrest

Emergency medical response systems should not require field personnel to transport every patient in cardiac arrest back to a hospital or to an ED. Transportation with continuing CPR is justified if interventions available in the ED cannot be performed in the out-of-hospital setting and they are indicated for special circumstances (ie, cardiopulmonary bypass or extracorporeal circulation for patients with severe hypothermia).

After OHCA with ROSC, transport the patient to an appropriate hospital with a comprehensive post–cardiac arrest treatment system of care that includes acute coronary interventions, neurologic care, critical care, and hypothermia. Transport the in-hospital post–cardiac arrest patient to an appropriate critical care unit capable of providing comprehensive post–cardiac arrest care.

Bradycardia Case

Introduction

This case discusses assessment and management of a *patient with symptomatic brady-cardia* (heart rate less than 50/min).

The cornerstones of managing bradycardia are to

- Differentiate between signs and symptoms that are caused by the slow rate versus those that are unrelated
- Correctly diagnose the presence and type of AV block
- Use atropine as the drug intervention of first choice
- Decide when to initiate transcutaneous pacing (TCP)
- Decide when to start epinephrine or dopamine to maintain heart rate and blood pressure
- Know when to call for expert consultation about complicated rhythm interpretation, drugs, or management decisions

In addition, you must know the techniques and cautions for using TCP.

Rhythms for Bradycardia

This case involves these ECG rhythms:

- Sinus bradycardia
- First-degree AV block
- Second-degree AV block
  - Type I (Wenckebach/Mobitz I)
  - Type II (Mobitz II)
- Third-degree AV block

You should know the major AV blocks because important treatment decisions are based on the type of block present (Figure 41). Complete AV block is generally the most important and clinically significant degree of block. Also, complete or third-degree AV block is the degree of block most likely to cause cardiovascular collapse and require immediate pacing. *Recognition of a symptomatic bradycardia due to AV block is a primary goal.* Recognition of the type of AV block is a secondary goal.

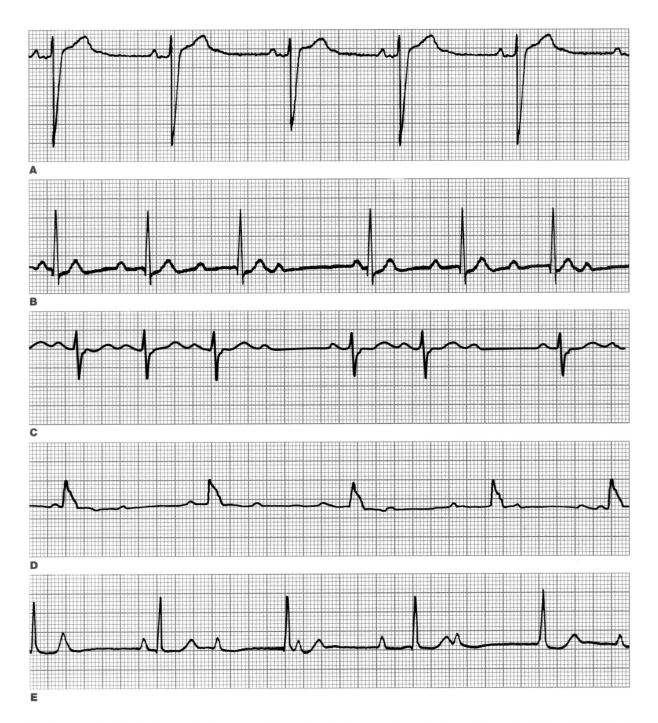

Figure 41. Examples of AV block. **A,** Sinus bradycardia with borderline first-degree AV block. **B,** Second-degree AV block type I. **C,** Second-degree AV block type II. **D,** Complete AV block with a ventricular escape pacemaker (wide QRS: 0.12 to 0.14 second). **E,** Third-degree AV block with a junctional escape pacemaker (narrow QRS: less than 0.12 second).

Drugs for Bradycardia

This case involves these drugs:

- Atropine
- Dopamine (infusion)
- Epinephrine (infusion)

Description of Bradycardia

Definitions

Definitions used in this case are as follows:

Term	Definition
Bradyarrhythmia or bradycardia*	Any rhythm disorder with a heart rate less than 60/min—eg, third-degree AV block—or sinus bradycardia. When bradycardia is the cause of symptoms, the rate is generally less than 50/min.
Symptomatic bradyarrhythmia	Signs and symptoms due to the slow heart rate

*For the purposes of this case, we will use the term *bradycardia* interchangeably with *bradyarrhythmia* unless specifically defined.

Symptomatic Bradycardia

Sinus bradycardia may have multiple causes. Some are physiologic and require no assessment or therapy. For example, a well-trained athlete may have a heart rate in the range of 40 to 50/min or occasionally lower.

In contrast, some patients have heart rates in the normal sinus range, but these heart rates are inappropriate or insufficient for them. This is called a *functional* or *relative* bradycardia. For example, a heart rate of 70/min may be relatively too slow for a patient in cardiogenic or septic shock.

This case will focus on the patient with a bradycardia and heart rate less than 50/min. Key to the case management is the determination of symptoms or signs due to the decreased heart rate. A symptomatic bradycardia exists clinically when 3 criteria are present:

1. The heart rate is slow.

2. The patient has symptoms.

3. The symptoms are due to the slow heart rate.

Signs and Symptoms

You must perform a focused history and physical examination to identify the signs and symptoms of a bradycardia.

Symptoms include chest discomfort or pain, shortness of breath, decreased level of consciousness, weakness, fatigue, light-headedness, dizziness, and presyncope or syncope.

Signs include hypotension, drop in blood pressure on standing (orthostatic hypotension), diaphoresis, pulmonary congestion on physical examination or chest x-ray, frank congestive heart failure or PE, and bradycardia-related (escape) frequent premature ventricular complexes or VT.

Managing Bradycardia: The Bradycardia Algorithm

Overview of the Algorithm

The Adult Bradycardia With a Pulse Algorithm (Figure 42) outlines the steps for assessment and management of a patient presenting with symptomatic bradycardia with pulse. Implementation of this algorithm begins with the identification of bradycardia (Step 1); the heart rate is less than 50/min. First steps include the components of the BLS Assessment and the Primary Assessment, such as supporting circulation and airway management, giving oxygen if indicated, monitoring the rhythm and vital signs, establishing IV access, and obtaining a 12-lead ECG if available (Step 2). In the differential diagnosis, you determine if the patient has signs or symptoms of poor perfusion and if these are caused by the bradycardia (Step 3).

The primary decision point in the algorithm is the determination of adequate perfusion. If the patient has adequate perfusion, you observe and monitor (Step 4). If the patient has poor perfusion, you administer atropine (Step 5). If atropine is ineffective, prepare for TCP or consider dopamine or epinephrine infusion (Step 5). If indicated, you prepare for transvenous pacing, search for and treat contributing causes, and seek expert consultation (Step 6).

The treatment sequence in the algorithm is determined by the severity of the patient's condition. You may need to implement multiple interventions simultaneously. If cardiac arrest develops, go to the Cardiac Arrest Algorithm.

Adult Bradycardia With a Pulse Algorithm

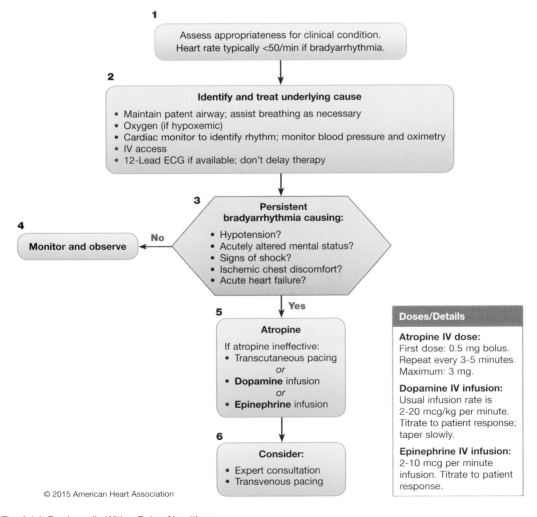

© 2015 American Heart Association

Figure 42. The Adult Bradycardia With a Pulse Algorithm.

Application of the Bradycardia Algorithm

Introduction

In this case, you have a patient presenting with symptoms of bradycardia. You conduct appropriate assessment and interventions as outlined in the Bradycardia Algorithm. At the same time, you are searching for and treating possible contributing factors.

Identification of Bradycardia

Identify whether the bradycardia is

- Present by definition, ie, heart rate less than 50/min
- Inadequate for the patient's condition (functional or relative)

Primary Assessment

Next, perform the Primary Assessment, including the following:

A	Maintain patent airway.
B	Assist breathing as needed; give oxygen in case of hypoxemia; monitor oxygen saturation.
C	Monitor blood pressure and heart rate; obtain and review a 12-lead ECG; establish IV access.
D	Conduct a problem-focused history and physical examination; search for and treat possible contributing factors.

Are Signs or Symptoms Caused by Bradycardia?

Step 3 prompts you to consider if the signs or symptoms of poor perfusion are caused by the bradycardia.

The key clinical questions are

- Are there "serious" signs or symptoms?
- Are the signs and symptoms related to the slow heart rate?

Look for adverse signs and symptoms of the bradycardia:

- Symptoms (eg, chest discomfort, shortness of breath, decreased level of consciousness, weakness, fatigue, light-headedness, dizziness, presyncope or syncope)
- Signs (eg, hypotension, congestive heart failure, ventricular arrhythmias related to the bradycardia)

Sometimes the "symptom" is not due to the bradycardia. For example, hypotension associated with bradycardia may be due to myocardial dysfunction rather than the bradycardia. Keep this in mind when you reassess the patient's response to treatment.

Critical Concepts

Bradycardia

The key clinical question is whether the bradycardia is causing the patient's symptoms or some other illness is causing the bradycardia.

Decision Point: Adequate Perfusion?

You must now decide if the patient has adequate or poor perfusion.

- If the patient has *adequate perfusion*, observe and monitor (Step 4).
- If the patient has *poor perfusion*, proceed to Step 5.

Treatment Sequence Summary

If the patient has poor perfusion secondary to bradycardia, the treatment sequence is as follows:

Give atropine as first-line treatment	Atropine 0.5 mg IV—may repeat to a total dose of 3 mg

If atropine is ineffective

Transcutaneous pacing	*or*	Dopamine 2 to 20 mcg/kg per minute (chronotropic or heart rate dose)
		Epinephrine 2 to 10 mcg/min

The treatment sequence is determined by the severity of the patient's clinical presentation. For patients with symptomatic bradycardia, move quickly through this sequence. These patients may be "pre–cardiac arrest" and may need multiple interventions simultaneously.

Avoid relying on atropine in type II second-degree or third-degree AV block or in patients with third-degree AV block with a new wide QRS complex where the location of the block is likely to be in infranodal tissue (such as in the bundle of His or more distal conduction system).

These bradyarrhythmias are not likely to be responsive to reversal of cholinergic effects by atropine and are preferably treated with TCP or β-adrenergic support as temporizing measures while the patient is prepared for transvenous pacing. Atropine administration should not delay implementation of external pacing or β-adrenergic infusion for patients with impending cardiac arrest.

Although not a first-line agent for treatment of symptomatic bradycardia, a β-adrenergic infusion (ie, dopamine, epinephrine) is an alternative when a bradyarrhythmia is unresponsive to, or inappropriate for, treatment with atropine, or as a temporizing measure while the patient is prepared for transvenous pacing.

No known vasopressor (epinephrine) increases survival from bradycardia. Because these medications can improve aortic diastolic blood pressure, coronary artery perfusion pressure, and the rate of ROSC, the AHA continues to recommend their use.

Alternative drugs may also be appropriate in special circumstances such as the overdose of a β-blocker or calcium channel blocker. Healthcare providers should not wait for a maximum dose of atropine if the patient is presenting with second-degree or third-degree block; rather, they may move to a second-line treatment after 2 to 3 doses of atropine.

Treatment Sequence: Atropine

In the absence of immediately reversible causes, atropine remains the first-line drug for acute symptomatic bradycardia. Atropine sulfate acts by reversing cholinergic-mediated decreases in the heart rate and AV node conduction. Dopamine and epinephrine may be successful as an alternative to TCP.

For bradycardia, give atropine 0.5 mg IV every 3 to 5 minutes to a total dose of 0.04 mg/kg (maximum total dose of 3 mg). Atropine doses of less than 0.5 mg may paradoxically result in further slowing of the heart rate.

Use atropine cautiously in the presence of acute coronary ischemia or MI. An atropine-mediated increase in heart rate may worsen ischemia or increase infarct size.

Do not rely on atropine in Mobitz type II second-degree or third-degree AV block or in patients with third-degree AV block with a new wide QRS complex.

Treatment Sequence: Pacing

TCP may be useful for treatment of symptomatic bradycardia. TCP is noninvasive and can be performed by ACLS providers.

Healthcare providers should consider immediate pacing in unstable patients with high-degree heart block when IV access is not available. It is reasonable for healthcare providers to initiate TCP in unstable patients who do not respond to atropine.

After initiation of pacing, confirm electrical and mechanical capture. Because heart rate is a major determinant of myocardial oxygen consumption, set the pacing rate to the lowest effective rate based on clinical assessment and symptom resolution. Reassess the patient for symptom improvement and hemodynamic stability. Give analgesics and sedatives for pain control. Note that many of these drugs may further decrease blood pressure and affect the patient's mental status. Try to identify and correct the cause of the bradycardia.

Some limitations apply. TCP can be painful and may not produce effective electrical and mechanical capture. If symptoms are not caused by the bradycardia, pacing may be ineffective despite capture. Because TCP is painful and not as reliable as transvenous pacing, it should be considered as an emergent bridge to transvenous pacing in patients with significant sinus bradycardia or AV block.

If you chose TCP as the second-line treatment and it is also ineffective (eg, inconsistent capture), begin an infusion of dopamine or epinephrine and prepare for possible transvenous pacing by obtaining expert consultation.

Foundational Facts

Sedation and Pacing

Most conscious patients should be given sedation before pacing. If the patient is in cardiovascular collapse or rapidly deteriorating, it may be necessary to start pacing without prior sedation, particularly if drugs for sedation are not immediately available. The clinician must evaluate the need for sedation in light of the patient's condition and need for immediate pacing. A review of the drugs used is beyond the scope of the ACLS Provider Course. The general approach could include the following:

- Give parenteral benzodiazepine for anxiety and muscle contractions.
- Give a parenteral narcotic for analgesia.
- Use a chronotropic infusion once available.
- Obtain expert consultation for transvenous pacing.

Treatment Sequence: Epinephrine, Dopamine

Although β-adrenergic agonists with rate-accelerating effects are not first-line agents for treatment of symptomatic bradycardia, they are alternatives to TCP or in special circumstances such as overdose with a β-blocker or calcium channel blocker.

Because epinephrine and dopamine are vasoconstrictors, as well as chronotropes, healthcare providers must assess the patient's intravascular volume status and avoid hypovolemia when using these drugs.

Both epinephrine and dopamine infusions may be used for patients with symptomatic bradycardia, particularly if associated with hypotension, for whom atropine may be inappropriate or after atropine fails.

Begin epinephrine infusion at a dose of 2 to 10 mcg/min and titrate to patient response.

Begin dopamine infusion at 2 to 20 mcg/kg per minute and titrate to patient response. At lower doses, dopamine has a more selective effect on inotropy and heart rate; at higher doses (greater than 10 mcg/kg per minute), it also has vasoconstrictive effects.

Next Actions

After consideration of the treatment sequence in Step 5, you may need to

- Prepare the patient for transvenous pacing
- Treat the contributing causes of the bradycardia
- Consider expert consultation—but do not delay treatment if the patient is unstable or potentially unstable

Transcutaneous Pacing

Introduction

A variety of devices can pace the heart by delivering an electrical stimulus, causing electrical depolarization and subsequent cardiac contraction. TCP delivers pacing impulses to the heart through the skin by use of cutaneous electrodes. Most manufacturers have added a pacing mode to manual defibrillators.

The ability to perform TCP is now often as close as the nearest defibrillator. Providers need to know the indications, techniques, and hazards for using TCP.

Indications

Indications for TCP are as follows:

- Hemodynamically unstable bradycardia (eg, hypotension, acutely altered mental status, signs of shock, ischemic chest discomfort, acute heart failure [AHF] hypotension)
- Unstable clinical condition likely due to the bradycardia
- For pacing readiness in the setting of AMI as follows:
  - Symptomatic sinus bradycardia
  - Mobitz type II second-degree AV block
  - Third-degree AV block
  - New left, right, or alternating bundle branch block or bifascicular block
- Bradycardia with symptomatic ventricular escape rhythms

Precautions

Precautions for TCP are as follows:

- TCP is contraindicated in severe hypothermia and is not recommended for asystole.
- Conscious patients require analgesia for discomfort unless delay for sedation will cause/contribute to deterioration.
- Do not assess the carotid pulse to confirm mechanical capture; electrical stimulation causes muscular jerking that may mimic the carotid pulse.

Technique

Perform TCP by following these steps:

Step	Action
1	Place pacing electrodes on the chest according to package instructions.
2	Turn the pacer on.
3	Set the demand rate to approximately 60/min. This rate can be adjusted up or down (based on patient clinical response) once pacing is established.
4	Set the current milliamperes output 2 mA above the dose at which consistent capture is observed (safety margin).

External pacemakers have either *fixed* rates (asynchronous mode) or *demand* rates.

Assess Response to Treatment

Rather than target a precise heart rate, the goal of therapy is to ensure improvement in clinical status (ie, signs and symptoms related to the bradycardia). Signs of hemodynamic impairment include hypotension, acutely altered mental status, signs of shock, ischemic chest discomfort, AHF, or other signs of shock related to the bradycardia. Start pacing at a rate of about 60/min. Once pacing is initiated, adjust the rate based on the patient's clinical response. Most patients will improve with a rate of 60 to 70/min if the symptoms are primarily due to the bradycardia.

Consider giving atropine before pacing in mildly symptomatic patients. Do not delay pacing for unstable patients, particularly those with high-degree AV block. Atropine may increase heart rate, improve hemodynamics, and eliminate the need for pacing. If atropine is ineffective or likely to be ineffective or if establishment of IV access or atropine administration is delayed, begin pacing as soon as it is available.

Patients with ACS should be paced at the lowest heart rate that allows clinical stability. Higher heart rates can worsen ischemia because heart rate is a major determinate of myocardial oxygen demand. Ischemia, in turn, can precipitate arrhythmias.

An alternative to pacing if symptomatic bradycardia is unresponsive to atropine is a chronotropic drug infusion to stimulate heart rate:

- Epinephrine: Initiate at 2 to 10 mcg/min and titrate to patient response
- Dopamine: Initiate at 2 to 20 mcg/kg per minute and titrate to patient response

Bradycardia With Escape Rhythms

A bradycardia may lead to secondary bradycardia-dependent ventricular rhythms. When the heart rate falls, an electrically unstable ventricular area may "escape" suppression by higher and faster pacemakers (eg, sinus node), especially in the setting of acute ischemia. These ventricular rhythms often fail to respond to drugs. With severe bradycardia, some patients will develop wide-complex ventricular beats that can precipitate VT or VF. Pacing may increase the heart rate and eliminate bradycardia-dependent ventricular rhythms. However, an accelerated idioventricular rhythm (sometimes called *AIVR*) may occur in the setting of inferior wall MI. This rhythm is usually stable and does not require pacing.

Patients with ventricular escape rhythms may have normal myocardium with disturbed conduction. After correction of electrolyte abnormalities or acidosis, rapid pacing can stimulate effective myocardial contractions until the conduction system recovers.

Standby Pacing

Several bradycardic rhythms in ACS are caused by acute ischemia of conduction tissue and pacing centers. Patients who are clinically stable may decompensate suddenly or become unstable over minutes to hours from worsening conduction abnormalities. These bradycardias may deteriorate to complete AV block and cardiovascular collapse.

Place TCP electrodes in anticipation of clinical deterioration in patients with acute myocardial ischemia or infarction associated with the following rhythms:

- Symptomatic sinus node dysfunction with severe and symptomatic sinus bradycardia
- Asymptomatic Mobitz type II second-degree AV block
- Asymptomatic third-degree AV block
- Newly acquired left, right, or alternating bundle branch block or bifascicular block in the setting of AMI

Tachycardia: Stable and Unstable

Introduction

If you are the team leader in this case, you will conduct the assessment and management of a *patient with a rapid, unstable heart rate*. You must be able to classify the tachycardia and implement appropriate interventions as outlined in the Tachycardia Algorithm. You will be evaluated on your knowledge of the factors involved in safe and effective synchronized cardioversion as well as your performance of the procedure.

Rhythms for Unstable Tachycardia

This case involves these ECG rhythms (examples in Figure 43):

- Sinus tachycardia
- Atrial fibrillation
- Atrial flutter
- Reentry supraventricular tachycardia (SVT)
- Monomorphic VT
- Polymorphic VT
- Wide-complex tachycardia of uncertain type

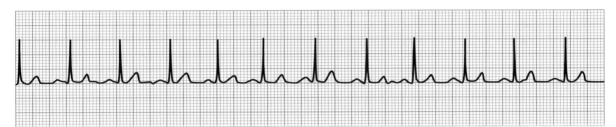

A

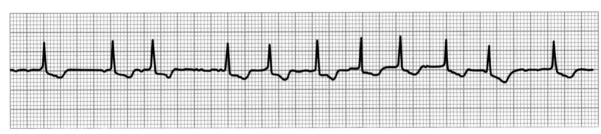

B

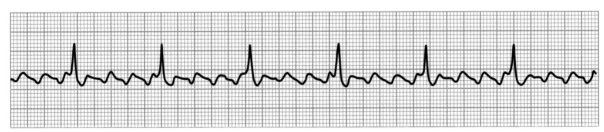

C

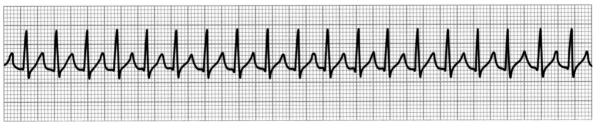

D

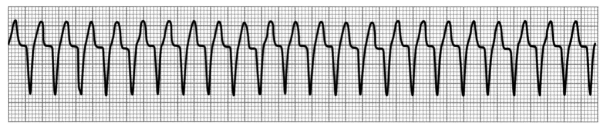

E

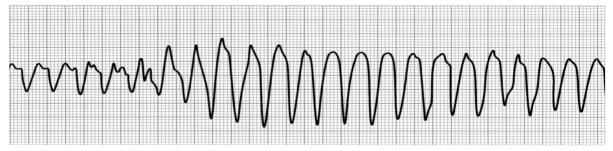

F

Figure 43. Examples of tachycardias. **A,** Sinus tachycardia. **B,** Atrial fibrillation. **C,** Atrial flutter. **D,** Supraventricular tachycardia. **E,** Monomorphic ventricular tachycardia. **F,** Polymorphic ventricular tachycardia.

Drugs for Unstable Tachycardia	Drugs are generally not used to manage patients with unstable tachycardia. Immediate cardioversion is recommended. Consider administering sedative drugs in the conscious patient. But do not delay immediate cardioversion in the unstable patient.

The Approach to Unstable Tachycardia

Introduction	A tachyarrhythmia (rhythm with heart rate greater than 100/min) has many potential causes and may be symptomatic or asymptomatic. The key to management of a patient with any tachycardia is to determine whether pulses are present. If pulses are present, determine whether the patient is stable or unstable and then provide treatment based on patient condition and rhythm. If the tachyarrhythmia is sinus tachycardia, conduct a diligent search for the cause of the tachycardia. Treatment and correction of this cause will improve the signs and symptoms.
Definitions	Definitions used in this case are as follows:

Term	Definition
Tachyarrhythmia, tachycardia*	Heart rate greater than 100/min
Symptomatic tachyarrhythmia	Signs and symptoms due to the rapid heart rate

*For the purposes of this case, we will use the term *tachycardia* interchangeably with *tachyarrhythmia.* Sinus tachycardia will be specifically indicated.

Pathophysiology of Unstable Tachycardia

Unstable tachycardia exists when the heart rate is too fast for the patient's clinical condition and the excessive heart rate causes symptoms or an unstable condition because the heart is

- *Beating so fast* that cardiac output is reduced; this can cause pulmonary edema, coronary ischemia, and hypotension with reduced blood flow to vital organs (eg, brain, kidneys)
- *Beating ineffectively* so that coordination between the atrium and ventricles or the ventricles themselves reduces cardiac output

Signs and Symptoms

Unstable tachycardia leads to serious signs and symptoms that include

- Hypotension
- Acutely altered mental status
- Signs of shock
- Ischemic chest discomfort
- AHF

Rapid Recognition Is the Key to Management

The 2 keys to management of patients with unstable tachycardia are

1. Rapid recognition that the patient is *significantly symptomatic* or even *unstable*

2. Rapid recognition that the *signs and symptoms are caused by the tachycardia*

You must quickly determine whether the patient's tachycardia is producing hemodynamic instability and serious signs and symptoms or whether the signs and symptoms (eg, the pain and distress of an AMI) are producing the tachycardia.

This determination can be difficult. Many experts suggest that when a heart rate is less than 150/min, it is unlikely that symptoms of instability are caused primarily by the tachycardia unless there is impaired ventricular function. A heart rate greater than 150/min is usually an inappropriate response to physiologic stress (eg, fever, dehydration) or other underlying conditions.

Severity

Assess for the presence or absence of signs and symptoms and for their severity. Frequent patient assessment is indicated.

Indications for Cardioversion

Rapid identification of symptomatic tachycardia will help you determine whether you should prepare for immediate cardioversion. For example:

- *Sinus tachycardia* is a physiologic response to extrinsic factors, such as fever, anemia, or hypotension/shock, which create the need for a compensatory and physiological increase in heart rate. There is usually a high degree of sympathetic tone and neurohormonal factors in these settings. Sinus tachycardia will not respond to cardioversion. In fact, if a shock is delivered, the heart rate often increases.
- If the patient with tachycardia is stable (ie, no serious signs related to the tachycardia), patients may await expert consultation because treatment has the potential for harm.
- *Atrial flutter* typically produces a heart rate of approximately 150/min (lower rates may be present in patients who have received antiarrhythmic therapy). Atrial flutter at this rate is often stable in the patient without heart or serious systemic disease.
- At rates greater than 150/min, symptoms are often present and cardioversion is often required if the patient is unstable.
- If the patient is seriously ill or has underlying cardiovascular disease, symptoms may be present at lower rates.

You must know when cardioversion is indicated, how to prepare the patient for it (including appropriate medication), and how to switch the defibrillator/monitor to operate as a cardioverter.

Managing Unstable Tachycardia: The Tachycardia Algorithm

Introduction

The Adult Tachycardia With a Pulse Algorithm simplifies initial management of tachycardia. The presence or absence of pulses is considered key to management of a patient with any tachycardia. If pulses are present, determine whether the patient is stable or unstable and then provide treatment based on the patient's condition and rhythm. If a pulseless tachycardia is present, then manage the patient according to the Cardiac Arrest Algorithm (Figure 31 in the section Managing VF/Pulseless VT: The Adult Cardiac Arrest Algorithm).

The ACLS provider should either be an expert or be able to obtain expert consultation. Actions in the steps require advanced knowledge of ECG rhythm interpretation and anti-arrhythmic therapy and are intended to be accomplished in the in-hospital setting with expert consultation available.

Overview

The Tachycardia Algorithm (Figure 44) outlines the steps for assessment and management of a patient presenting with symptomatic tachycardia with pulses. Implementation of this algorithm begins with the identification of tachycardia with pulses (Step 1). If a tachycardia and a pulse are present, perform assessment and management steps guided by the BLS Assessment and the Primary and Secondary Assessments (Step 2). The key in this assessment is to decide if the tachycardia is stable or unstable.

If signs and symptoms persist despite provision of supplementary oxygen and support of airway and circulation and if significant signs or symptoms are due to the tachycardia (Step 3), then the tachycardia is unstable and immediate synchronized cardioversion is indicated (Step 4).

If the patient is stable, you will evaluate the ECG, and determine if the QRS complex is wide or narrow and regular or irregular (Step 5). The treatment of stable tachycardia is presented in the next case (Step 6).

A precise diagnosis of the rhythm (eg, reentry SVT, atrial flutter) may not be possible at this time.

Foundational Facts

Serious or Significant Symptoms

Unstable Condition

Intervention is determined by the presence of significant symptoms or by an unstable condition resulting from the tachycardia.*

Serious symptoms and signs include

- Hypotension
- Acutely altered mental status
- Signs of shock
- Ischemic chest discomfort
- AHF

*Ventricular rates less than 150/min usually do not cause serious signs or symptoms.

Adult Tachycardia With a Pulse Algorithm

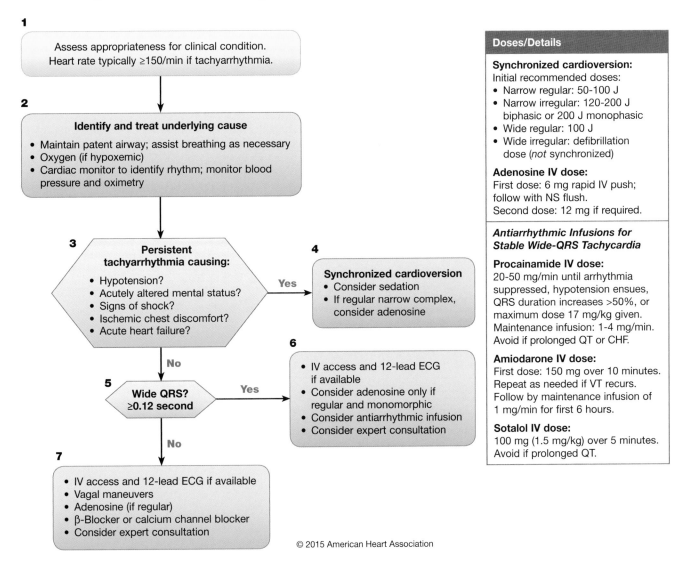

1

Assess appropriateness for clinical condition.
Heart rate typically ≥150/min if tachyarrhythmia.

2

Identify and treat underlying cause

- Maintain patent airway; assist breathing as necessary
- Oxygen (if hypoxemic)
- Cardiac monitor to identify rhythm; monitor blood pressure and oximetry

3

Persistent tachyarrhythmia causing:

- Hypotension?
- Acutely altered mental status?
- Signs of shock?
- Ischemic chest discomfort?
- Acute heart failure?

Yes

4

Synchronized cardioversion

- Consider sedation
- If regular narrow complex, consider adenosine

No

5

Wide QRS?
≥0.12 second

Yes

6

- IV access and 12-lead ECG if available
- Consider adenosine only if regular and monomorphic
- Consider antiarrhythmic infusion
- Consider expert consultation

No

7

- IV access and 12-lead ECG if available
- Vagal maneuvers
- Adenosine (if regular)
- β-Blocker or calcium channel blocker
- Consider expert consultation

Doses/Details

Synchronized cardioversion:
Initial recommended doses:
- Narrow regular: 50-100 J
- Narrow irregular: 120-200 J biphasic or 200 J monophasic
- Wide regular: 100 J
- Wide irregular: defibrillation dose (*not* synchronized)

Adenosine IV dose:
First dose: 6 mg rapid IV push; follow with NS flush.
Second dose: 12 mg if required.

Antiarrhythmic Infusions for Stable Wide-QRS Tachycardia

Procainamide IV dose:
20-50 mg/min until arrhythmia suppressed, hypotension ensues, QRS duration increases >50%, or maximum dose 17 mg/kg given. Maintenance infusion: 1-4 mg/min. Avoid if prolonged QT or CHF.

Amiodarone IV dose:
First dose: 150 mg over 10 minutes. Repeat as needed if VT recurs. Follow by maintenance infusion of 1 mg/min for first 6 hours.

Sotalol IV dose:
100 mg (1.5 mg/kg) over 5 minutes. Avoid if prolonged QT.

© 2015 American Heart Association

Figure 44. The Adult Tachycardia With a Pulse Algorithm.

Summary

Your assessment and management of this patient will be guided by the following key questions presented in the Tachycardia Algorithm:

- Are symptoms present or absent?
- Is the patient stable or unstable?
- Is the QRS narrow or wide?
- Is the rhythm regular or irregular?
- Is the QRS monomorphic or polymorphic?

Your answers to these questions will determine the next appropriate steps.

Application of the Tachycardia Algorithm to the Unstable Patient

Introduction

In this case, you have a patient with tachycardia and a pulse. You conduct the steps outlined in the Tachycardia Algorithm to evaluate and manage the patient.

Assess Appropriateness for Clinical Condition

- Tachycardia is defined as an arrhythmia with a rate greater than 100/min.
- The rate takes on clinical significance at its greater extremes and is more likely attributable to an arrhythmia rate of 150/min or greater.
- It is unlikely that symptoms of instability are caused primarily by the tachycardia when the heart rate is less than 150/min unless there is impaired ventricular function.

Identify and Treat the Underlying Cause

Use the BLS, Primary, and Secondary Assessments to guide your approach.

- Look for signs of increased work of breathing (tachypnea, intercostal retractions, suprasternal retractions, paradoxical abdominal breathing) and hypoxemia as determined by pulse oximetry.
- Give oxygen, if indicated, and monitor oxygen saturation.
- Obtain an ECG to identify the rhythm.
- Evaluate blood pressure.
- Establish IV access.
- Identify and treat reversible causes.

If symptoms persist despite support of adequate oxygenation and ventilation, proceed to Step 3.

Critical Concepts

Unstable Patients

- Healthcare providers should obtain a 12-lead ECG early in the assessment to better define the rhythm.
- However, **unstable patients require immediate cardioversion.**
- Do not delay immediate cardioversion for acquisition of the 12-lead ECG if the patient is unstable.

Decision Point: Is the Persistent Tachyarrhythmia Causing Significant Signs or Symptoms?

Assess the patient's degree of instability and determine if the instability is related to the tachycardia.

Unstable

If the patient demonstrates rate-related cardiovascular compromise with signs and symptoms such as hypotension, acutely altered mental status, signs of shock, ischemic chest discomfort, AHF, or other signs of shock suspected to be due to a tachyarrhythmia, proceed to immediate synchronized cardioversion (Step 4).

Serious signs and symptoms are unlikely if the ventricular rate is less than 150/min in patients with a healthy heart. However, if the patient is seriously ill or has significant underlying heart disease or other conditions, symptoms may be present at a lower heart rate.

Stable

If the patient does not have rate-related cardiovascular compromise, proceed to Step 5. The healthcare provider has time to obtain a 12-lead ECG, evaluate the rhythm, determine the width of the QRS, and determine treatment options. Stable patients may await expert consultation because treatment has the potential for harm.

Foundational Facts

Treatment Based on Type of Tachycardia

You may not always be able to distinguish between supraventricular and ventricular rhythms. Most wide-complex (broad-complex) tachycardias are ventricular in origin (especially if the patient has underlying heart disease or is older). If the patient is pulse-less, treat the rhythm as VF and follow the Cardiac Arrest Algorithm.

If the patient has a wide-complex tachycardia and is unstable, assume it is VT until proven otherwise. The amount of energy required for cardioversion of VT is determined by the morphologic characteristics.

- If the patient is unstable but has a pulse with regular uniform wide-complex VT (*mono-morphic VT*):
  - Treat with synchronized cardioversion and an initial shock of 100 J (monophasic waveform).
  - If there is no response to the first shock, increasing the dose in a stepwise fashion is reasonable.*
- Arrhythmias with a polymorphic QRS appearance (*polymorphic VT*), such as torsades de pointes, will usually not permit synchronization. If the patient has *polymorphic VT*:
  - Treat as VF with high-energy unsynchronized shocks (eg, defibrillation doses).

If there is any doubt about whether an unstable patient has monomorphic or polymor-phic VT, do not delay treatment for further rhythm analysis. Provide high-energy, unsyn-chronized shocks.

*No studies that addressed this issue had been identified at the time that the manuscript for the *2015 AHA Guidelines Update for CPR and ECC* was in preparation. Thus, this recommendation represents expert opinion.

Perform Immediate Synchronized Cardioversion

- If possible, establish IV access before cardioversion and administer sedation if the patient is conscious.
- Do not delay cardioversion if the patient is extremely unstable.

Further information about cardioversion appears below.

If the patient with a regular narrow-complex SVT or a monomorphic wide-complex tachy-cardia is not hypotensive, healthcare providers may administer adenosine while preparing for synchronized cardioversion.

If cardiac arrest develops, see the Cardiac Arrest Algorithm.

Determine the Width of the QRS Complex

- If the width of the QRS complex is 0.12 second or more, go to Step 6.
- If the width of the QRS complex is less than 0.12 second, go to Step 7.

Cardioversion

Introduction

You must know when cardioversion is indicated and what type of shock to administer. Before cardioversion, establish IV access and sedate the responsive patient if possible, but do not delay cardioversion in the unstable or deteriorating patient.

This section discusses the following important concepts about cardioversion:

- The difference between unsynchronized and synchronized shocks
- Potential challenges to delivery of synchronized shocks
- Energy doses for specific rhythms

Unsynchronized vs Synchronized Shocks

Modern defibrillator/cardioverters are capable of delivering 2 types of shocks:

- Unsynchronized shocks
- Synchronized shocks

An *unsynchronized* shock simply means that the electrical shock will be delivered as soon as the operator pushes the shock button to discharge the device. Thus, the shock may fall randomly anywhere within the cardiac cycle. *These shocks should use higher energy levels than synchronized cardioversion.*

Synchronized cardioversion uses a sensor to deliver a shock that is synchronized with a peak of the QRS complex (eg, the highest point of the R wave). When this option (the "sync" option) is engaged, the operator presses the shock button to deliver a shock. There will likely be a delay before the defibrillator/cardioverter delivers a shock because the device will synchronize shock delivery with the peak of the R wave in the patient's QRS complex. This synchronization may require analysis of several complexes. Synchronization avoids the delivery of a shock during cardiac repolarization (represented on the surface ECG as the T wave), a period of vulnerability in which a shock can precipitate VF. Synchronized cardioversion uses a lower energy level than attempted defibrillation. Low-energy shocks should always be delivered as synchronized shocks to avoid precipitating VF.

Potential Problems With Synchronization

In theory, synchronization is simple. The operator pushes the sync control on the face of the defibrillator/cardioverter. In practice, however, there are potential problems. For example:

- If the R-wave peaks of a tachycardia are undifferentiated or of low amplitude, the monitor sensors may be unable to identify an R-wave peak and therefore will not deliver the shock.
- Many cardioverters will not synchronize through the handheld quick-look paddles. An unwary practitioner may try to synchronize—unsuccessfully in that the machine will not discharge—and may not recognize the problem.
- Synchronization can take extra time (eg, if it is necessary to attach electrodes or if the operator is unfamiliar with the equipment).

Recommendations

When to Use Synchronized Shocks

Synchronized shocks are recommended for patients with

- Unstable SVT
- Unstable atrial fibrillation
- Unstable atrial flutter
- Unstable regular monomorphic tachycardia with pulses

When to Use Unsynchronized Shocks

Unsynchronized high-energy shocks are recommended

- For a patient who is pulseless
- For a patient demonstrating clinical deterioration (in prearrest), such as those with severe shock or polymorphic VT, when you think a delay in converting the rhythm will result in cardiac arrest
- When you are unsure whether monomorphic or polymorphic VT is present in the unstable patient

Should the shock cause VF (occurring in only a very small minority of patients despite the theoretical risk), immediately attempt defibrillation.

Energy Doses for Cardioversion

Select the energy dose for the specific type of rhythm.

For unstable atrial fibrillation:

- Monophasic cardioversion: Deliver an initial 200-J synchronized shock.
- Biphasic cardioversion: Deliver an initial 120- to 200-J synchronized shock.
- In either case, increase the energy dose in a stepwise fashion for any subsequent cardioversion attempts.

A dose of 120 to 200 J is reasonable with a biphasic waveform. Escalate the second and subsequent shock dose as needed.

Cardioversion of atrial flutter and SVT generally require less energy. An initial energy dose of 50 to 100 J with a monophasic or biphasic waveform is often sufficient.

Monomorphic VT (regular form and rate) with a pulse responds well to monophasic or biphasic waveform cardioversion (synchronized) shocks at an initial dose of 100 J. If there is no response to the first shock, increase the dose in a stepwise fashion. No studies were identified that addressed this issue. Thus, this recommendation represents expert opinion.

Synchronized Cardioversion Technique

Introduction

Synchronized cardioversion is the treatment of choice when a patient has a symptomatic (unstable) reentry SVT or VT with pulses. It is also recommended to treat unstable atrial fibrillation and unstable atrial flutter.

Cardioversion is unlikely to be effective for treatment of junctional tachycardia or ectopic or multifocal atrial tachycardia because these rhythms have an automatic focus arising from cells that are spontaneously depolarizing at a rapid rate. Delivery of a shock generally cannot stop these rhythms and may actually increase the rate of the tachyarrhythmia.

In synchronized cardioversion, shocks are administered through adhesive electrodes or handheld paddles. *You will need to place the defibrillator/monitor in synchronized (sync) mode.* The sync mode is designed to deliver energy just after the R wave of the QRS complex.

Technique

Follow these steps to perform synchronized cardioversion. Modify the steps for your specific device.

Step	Action
1	Sedate all conscious patients unless unstable or deteriorating rapidly.
2	Turn on the defibrillator (monophasic or biphasic).
3	Attach monitor leads to the patient ("white to right, red to ribs, what's left over to the left shoulder") and ensure proper display of the patient's rhythm. Position adhesive electrode (conductor) pads on the patient.
4	Press the sync control button to engage the synchronization mode.
5	Look for markers on the R wave indicating sync mode.
6	Adjust monitor gain if necessary until sync markers occur with each R wave.
7	Select the appropriate energy level. Deliver monophasic synchronized shocks in the following sequence: *table below* *Biphasic waveforms using lower energy are acceptable if documented to be clinically equivalent or superior to reports of monophasic shock success. Extrapolation from elective cardioversion of atrial fibrillation supports an initial biphasic dose of 120 to 200 J with escalation as needed. Consult the device manufacturer for specific recommendations.
8	Announce to team members: "Charging defibrillator—stand clear!"
9	Press the charge button.
10	Clear the patient when the defibrillator is charged. (See "Foundational Facts: Clearing for Defibrillation" in the VF/Pulseless VT Case.)
11	Press the shock button(s).
12	Check the monitor. If tachycardia persists, increase the energy level (joules) according to the Electrical Cardioversion Algorithm (see Supplementary Materials on the ACLS Student Website; **www.heart.org/eccstudent**).
13	Activate the sync mode after delivery of each synchronized shock. *Most defibrillators default back to the unsynchronized mode after delivery of a synchronized shock.* This default allows an immediate shock if cardioversion produces VF.

If	Initial Dose*
Unstable atrial fibrillation	200 J
Unstable monomorphic VT	100 J
Other unstable SVT/atrial flutter	50 to 100 J
Polymorphic VT (irregular form and rate) and unstable	Treat as VF with high-energy shock (defibrillation doses)

Stable Tachycardias

This case reviews assessment and management of a *stable patient (ie, no serious signs related to the tachycardia) with a rapid heart rate.* Patients with heart rates greater than 100/min have a tachyarrhythmia or tachycardia. In this case, we will use the terms *tachycardia* and *tachyarrhythmia* interchangeably. Note that sinus tachycardia is excluded from the treatment algorithm. Sinus tachycardia is almost always physiologic, developing in response to a compromise in stroke volume or a condition that requires an increase in cardiac output (eg, fever, hypovolemia). Treatment involves identification and correction of that underlying problem.

You must be able to classify the type of tachycardia (wide or narrow; regular or irregular) and implement appropriate interventions as outlined in the Tachycardia Algorithm. During this case you will

- Perform initial assessment and management
- Treat regular narrow-complex rhythms (except sinus tachycardia) with vagal maneuvers and adenosine

If the rhythm does not convert, you will monitor the patient and transport or obtain expert consultation. If the patient becomes clinically unstable, you will prepare for immediate unsynchronized shock or synchronized cardioversion as discussed in the Unstable Tachycardia Case.

Rhythms for Stable Tachycardia

Tachycardias can be classified in several ways based on the appearance of the QRS complex, heart rate, and whether they are regular or irregular:

- Narrow–QRS complex (SVT) tachycardias (QRS less than 0.12 second) in order of frequency
  - Sinus tachycardia
  - Atrial fibrillation
  - Atrial flutter
  - AV nodal reentry
- Wide–QRS complex tachycardias (QRS 0.12 second or more)
  - Monomorphic VT
  - Polymorphic VT
  - SVT with aberrancy
- Regular or irregular tachycardias
  - Irregular narrow-complex tachycardias are probably atrial fibrillation

Drugs for Stable Tachycardia

This case involves the following drug:

- Adenosine

Several agents are also used to provide analgesia and sedation during electrical cardioversion. These agents are not covered in the ACLS Provider Course.

Approach to Stable Tachycardia

Introduction

In this case, a stable tachycardia refers to a condition in which the patient has

- A heart rate greater than 100/min
- No significant signs or symptoms caused by the increased rate
- An underlying cardiac electrical abnormality that generates the rhythm

Questions to Determine Classification

Classification of the tachycardia depends on the careful clinical evaluation of these questions:

- Are symptoms present or absent?
- Are symptoms due to the tachycardia?
- Is the patient stable or unstable?
- Is the QRS complex narrow or wide?
- Is the rhythm regular or irregular?
- Is the QRS monomorphic or polymorphic?
- Is the rhythm sinus tachycardia?

The answers guide subsequent diagnosis and treatment.

Foundational Facts

Understanding Sinus Tachycardia

- Sinus tachycardia is a heart rate that is greater than 100/min and is generated by sinus node discharge. The heart rate in sinus tachycardia does not exceed 220/min and is age-related. Sinus tachycardia usually does not exceed 120 to 130/min, and it has a gradual onset and gradual termination. Reentry SVT has an abrupt onset and termination.

- Sinus tachycardia is caused by *external influences* on the heart, such as fever, anemia, hypotension, blood loss, or exercise. These are systemic conditions, not cardiac conditions. Sinus tachycardia is a regular rhythm, although the rate may be slowed by vagal maneuvers. Cardioversion is contraindicated.

- β-Blockers may cause clinical deterioration if the cardiac output falls when *a compensatory* tachycardia is blocked. This is because cardiac output is determined by the volume of blood ejected by the ventricles with each contraction (stroke volume) and the heart rate.

Cardiac output (CO) = Stroke volume (SV) × Heart rate

- If a condition such as a large AMI limits ventricular function (severe heart failure or cardiogenic shock), the heart compensates by increasing the heart rate. If you attempt to reduce the heart rate in patients with a compensatory tachycardia, cardiac output will fall and the patient's condition will likely deteriorate.

In sinus tachycardia, the goal is to identify and treat the underlying systemic cause.

Managing Stable Tachycardia: The Tachycardia Algorithm

Introduction

As noted in the Unstable Tachycardia Case, the key to management of a patient with any tachycardia is to determine whether pulses are present, and if pulses are present, to determine whether the patient is stable or unstable and then to provide treatment based on patient condition and rhythm. If the patient is pulseless, manage the patient according to the Cardiac Arrest Algorithm (Figure 31 in the section Managing VF/Pulseless VT: The Adult Cardiac Arrest Algorithm). If the patient has pulses, manage the patient according to the Tachycardia Algorithm (Figure 44).

Overview	If a tachycardia and a pulse are present, perform assessment and management steps guided by the BLS Assessment and the Primary and Secondary Assessments. Determine if significant symptoms or signs are present and if these symptoms and signs are due to the tachycardia. This will direct you to either the *stable (Steps 5 through 7)* or *unstable (Step 4)* section of the algorithm. • If significant signs or symptoms are due to the tachycardia, then the tachycardia is *unstable* and immediate cardioversion is indicated (see the Unstable Tachycardia Case). • If the patient develops *pulseless VT,* deliver unsynchronized high-energy shocks (defibrillation energy) and follow the Cardiac Arrest Algorithm. • If the patient has *polymorphic VT,* treat the rhythm as VF and deliver high-energy unsynchronized shocks (ie, defibrillation energy). In this case, the patient is *stable,* and you will manage according to the stable section of the Tachycardia Algorithm (Figure 44). A precise identification of the rhythm (eg, reentry SVT, atrial flutter) may not be possible at this time.

Application of the Tachycardia Algorithm to the Stable Patient

Introduction	In this case, a *patient has stable tachycardia with a pulse.* Conduct the steps outlined in the Tachycardia Algorithm to evaluate and manage the patient.
Patient Assessment	Step 1 directs you to assess the patient's condition. Typically, a heart rate greater than 150/min at rest is due to tachyarrhythmias other than sinus tachycardia.
BLS and ACLS Assessments	Using the BLS, Primary, and Secondary Assessments to guide your approach, evaluate the patient and do the following as necessary: • Look for signs of increased work of breathing and hypoxia as determined by pulse oximetry. • Give oxygen; monitor oxygen saturation. • Support the airway, breathing, and circulation. • Obtain an ECG to identify the rhythm; check blood pressure. • Identify and treat reversible causes. If symptoms persist, proceed to Step 3.
Decision Point: Stable or Unstable	*Unstable* If the patient is *unstable* with signs or symptoms as a result of the tachycardia (eg, hypotension, acutely altered mental status, signs of shock, ischemic chest discomfort, or AHF), go to Step 4 (perform immediate synchronized cardioversion). See the Unstable Tachycardia Case. *Stable* If the patient is stable, go to Step 5.
IV Access and 12-Lead ECG	If the patient with tachycardia is *stable* (ie, no serious signs or symptoms related to the tachycardia), you have time to evaluate the rhythm and decide on treatment options. Establish IV access if not already obtained. Obtain a 12-lead ECG (when available) or rhythm strip to determine if the QRS is narrow (less than 0.12 second) or wide (0.12 second or more).

Decision Point: Narrow or Wide

The path of treatment is now determined by whether the QRS is wide (Step 6) or narrow (Step 7), and whether the rhythm is regular or irregular. If a monomorphic wide-complex rhythm is present and the patient is stable, expert consultation is advised. Polymorphic wide-complex tachycardia should be treated with immediate unsynchronized cardioversion.

Foundational Facts

Treating Tachycardia

- You may not always be able to distinguish between supraventricular (aberrant) and ventricular wide-complex rhythms. If you are unsure, be aware that most wide-complex (broad-complex) tachycardias are *ventricular* in origin.
- If a patient is *pulseless*, follow the Cardiac Arrest Algorithm.
- If a patient becomes *unstable*, do not delay treatment for further rhythm analysis. For *stable* patients with wide-complex tachycardias, transport and monitor or consult an expert, because treatment has the potential for harm.

Wide-Complex Tachycardias

Wide-complex tachycardias are defined as a QRS of 0.12 second or more. *Consider expert consultation.*

The most common forms of life-threatening wide-complex tachycardias likely to deteriorate to VF are

- Monomorphic VT
- Polymorphic VT

Determine if the rhythm is regular or irregular.

- A regular wide-complex tachycardia is presumed to be VT or SVT with aberrancy.
- An irregular wide-complex tachycardia may be atrial fibrillation with aberrancy, pre-excited atrial fibrillation (atrial fibrillation using an accessory pathway for antegrade conduction), or polymorphic VT/torsades de pointes. These are advanced rhythms requiring additional expertise or expert consultation.

If the rhythm is likely VT or SVT in a stable patient, treat based on the algorithm for that rhythm.

If the rhythm etiology cannot be determined and is regular in its rate and monomorphic, recent evidence suggests that IV adenosine is relatively safe for both treatment and diagnosis. IV antiarrhythmic drugs may be effective. We recommend procainamide, amiodarone, or sotalol. See the right column of the Tachycardia Algorithm (Figure 44) for recommended doses.

In the case of irregular wide-complex tachycardia, management focuses on control of the rapid ventricular rate (rate control), conversion of hemodynamically unstable atrial fibrillation to sinus rhythm (rhythm control), or both. Expert consultation is advised.

Caution

Drugs to Avoid in Patients With Irregular Wide-Complex Tachycardia

Avoid AV nodal blocking agents such as adenosine, calcium channel blockers, digoxin, and possibly β-blockers in patients with pre-excitation atrial fibrillation, because these drugs may cause a paradoxical increase in the ventricular response.

Narrow QRS, Regular Rhythm

The therapy for narrow QRS with regular rhythm is

- Attempt vagal maneuvers
- Give adenosine

Vagal maneuvers and adenosine are the preferred initial interventions for terminating narrow-complex tachycardias that are symptomatic (but stable) and supraventricular in origin (SVT). Vagal maneuvers alone (Valsalva maneuver or carotid sinus massage) will terminate about 25% of SVTs. Adenosine is required for the remainder.

If SVT does not respond to vagal maneuvers:

- Give **adenosine** 6 mg as a rapid IV push in a large (eg, antecubital) vein over 1 second. Follow with a 20 mL saline flush and elevate the arm immediately.
- If SVT does not convert within 1 to 2 minutes, give a second dose of adenosine 12 mg rapid IV push following the same procedure above.

Adenosine increases AV block and will terminate approximately 90% of reentry arrhythmias within 2 minutes. Adenosine will not terminate atrial flutter or atrial fibrillation but will slow AV conduction, allowing for identification of flutter or fibrillation waves.

Adenosine is safe and effective in pregnancy. Adenosine does, however, have several important drug interactions. Larger doses may be required for patients with significant blood levels of theophylline, caffeine, or theobromine. The initial dose should be reduced to 3 mg in patients taking dipyridamole or carbamazepine. There have been recent case reports of prolonged asystole after adenosine administration to patients with transplanted hearts or after central venous administration, so lower doses such as 3 mg may be considered in these situations.

Adenosine may cause bronchospasm; therefore, adenosine should generally not be given to patients with asthma or chronic obstructive pulmonary disease, particularly if patients are actively bronchospastic.

If the rhythm converts with adenosine, it is probable reentry SVT. Observe for recurrence. Treat recurrence with adenosine or longer-acting AV nodal blocking agents such as the non-dihydropyridine calcium channel blockers (verapamil and diltiazem) or β-blockers. Typically, you should obtain expert consultation if the tachycardia recurs.

If the rhythm does not convert with adenosine, it is possible atrial flutter, ectopic atrial tachycardia, or junctional tachycardia. Obtain expert consultation about diagnosis and treatment.

Caution

What to Avoid With AV Nodal Blocking Agents

AV nodal blocking drugs should not be used for pre-excited atrial fibrillation or flutter. Treatment with an AV nodal blocking agent is unlikely to slow the ventricular rate and in some instances may accelerate the ventricular response. Caution is advised when combining AV nodal blocking agents that have a longer duration of action, such as calcium channel blockers or β-blockers, because their actions may overlap if given serially, which can provoke profound bradycardia.

Tachycardia Algorithm: Advanced Management Steps

Some ACLS providers may be familiar with the differential diagnosis and therapy of stable tachycardias that do not respond to initial treatment. The basic ACLS provider is expected to recognize a stable narrow-complex or wide-complex tachycardia and classify the rhythm as regular or irregular. Regular narrow-complex tachycardias may be treated initially with vagal maneuvers and adenosine. If these are unsuccessful, the ACLS provider should transport or *seek expert consultation*.

If ACLS providers have experience with the differential diagnosis and therapy of stable tachycardias beyond initial management, the Tachycardia Algorithm lists additional steps and pharmacologic agents used in the treatment of these arrhythmias, both for rate control and for termination of the arrhythmia.

If at any point you become uncertain or uncomfortable during the treatment of a stable patient, seek expert consultation. The treatment of stable patients may await expert consultation because treatment has the potential for harm.

Immediate Post–Cardiac Arrest Care Case

Introduction

There is increasing recognition that systematic post–cardiac arrest care after ROSC can improve the likelihood of patient survival with good quality of life. Positive correlations have been observed between the likelihood of survival and the number of cardiac arrest cases treated at any individual hospital.[41,42] Studies show most deaths occur during the first 24 hours after resuscitation from cardiac arrest.[43,44] Post–cardiac arrest care has a significant potential to reduce early mortality caused by hemodynamic instability and later morbidity and mortality caused by multiorgan failure and brain injury.[45,46]

There is a growing body of research focused on the identification and optimization of practices that improve outcomes of patients who achieve ROSC after cardiac arrest.[47] Mere restoration of blood pressure and gas exchange does not ensure survival and functional recovery. Significant cardiovascular dysfunction can develop after ROSC that requires active support of blood flow and ventilation, including intravascular volume expansion, vasoactive and inotropic drugs, and invasive devices. Targeted temperature management (TTM) and treatment of the underlying cause of cardiac arrest impact survival and neurologic outcome. Hemodynamic optimization protocols have been introduced as part of a bundle of care to improve survival.[48-50] The data suggest that proactive management of post–cardiac arrest physiology can improve outcomes by ensuring organ oxygenation and perfusion and by avoiding and managing complications.

This case focuses on the management and optimization of cardiopulmonary function and perfusion of vital organs after ROSC.

To ensure the success of post–cardiac arrest care, healthcare providers must

- Optimize the patient's hemodynamic and ventilation status
- Initiate TTM
- Provide immediate coronary reperfusion with PCI
- Provide neurologic care and prognostication and other structured interventions

In this case, you will have an opportunity to use the 12-lead ECG while using the assessment and action skills typically performed after ROSC.

Rhythms for Post–Cardiac Arrest Care

You will need to recognize the following rhythms:

- Rate—too fast or too slow
- Width of QRS complexes—wide versus narrow

Drugs for Post–Cardiac Arrest Care

This case involves these drugs:

- Epinephrine infusion
- Dopamine infusion
- Norepinephrine infusions

Multiple System Approach to Post–Cardiac Arrest Care

A comprehensive, structured, multidisciplinary system of care should be implemented in a consistent manner for the treatment of post–cardiac arrest patients. Programs should include TTM, optimization of hemodynamics and gas exchange, immediate coronary reperfusion when indicated for restoration of coronary blood flow with PCI, neurologic diagnosis, critical care management, and prognostication.

Clinicians should treat the precipitating cause of cardiac arrest after ROSC and initiate or request studies that will further aid in evaluation of the patient. It is essential to identify and treat any cardiac, electrolyte, toxicologic, pulmonary, and neurologic precipitants of arrest.

Overview of Post–Cardiac Arrest Care

Providers should ensure an adequate airway and support breathing immediately after ROSC. Unconscious patients usually require an advanced airway for mechanical support of breathing. Providers should also elevate the head of the bed 30° if tolerated to reduce the incidence of cerebral edema, aspiration, and ventilatory-associated pneumonia. Proper placement of an advanced airway, particularly during patient transport, should be monitored by waveform capnography as described in the *2015 AHA Guidelines Update for CPR and ECC*. Oxygenation of the patient should be monitored continuously with pulse oximetry.

Although 100% oxygen may have been used during initial resuscitation, providers should titrate inspired oxygen to the lowest level required to achieve an arterial oxygen saturation of 94% to 99% to avoid potential oxygen toxicity. Hyperventilation is common after cardiac arrest and should be avoided because of the potential for adverse hemodynamic effects. Hyperventilation increases intrathoracic pressure, which decreases preload and lowers cardiac output. The decrease in $PaCO_2$ seen with hyperventilation can also decrease cerebral blood flow directly. Ventilation should be started at 10/min and titrated to achieve a $PETCO_2$ of 35 to 40 mm Hg or a $PaCO_2$ of 40 to 45 mm Hg.

Healthcare providers should frequently reassess vital signs and monitor for recurrent cardiac arrhythmias by using continuous ECG monitoring. If the patient is hypotensive (SBP less than 90 mm Hg), fluid boluses can be administered. If TTM is indicated, cold fluids may be helpful for initial induction of hypothermia. If the patient's volume status is adequate, infusions of vasoactive agents may be initiated and titrated to achieve a minimum SBP of 90 mm Hg or greater or a mean arterial pressure of 65 mm Hg or more. Some advocate higher mean arterial pressures to promote cerebral blood flow.

Brain injury and cardiovascular instability are the major factors that determine survival after cardiac arrest.[51] Because TTM is currently the only intervention demonstrated to improve neurologic recovery, it should be considered for any patient who is comatose and unresponsive to verbal commands after ROSC. The patient should be transported to a location that reliably provides this therapy in addition to coronary reperfusion (eg, PCI) and other goal-directed postarrest care therapies.

Clinicians should treat the precipitating cause of cardiac arrest after ROSC and initiate or request studies that will further aid in evaluation of the patient. It is essential to identify and treat any cardiac, electrolyte, toxicologic, pulmonary, and neurologic precipitants of arrest. Overall, the most common cause of cardiac arrest is cardiovascular disease and associated coronary ischemia.[52,53] Therefore, a 12-lead ECG should be obtained as soon as possible to detect ST elevation or LBBB. Coronary angiography should be performed emergently (rather than later in the hospital stay or not at all) for OHCA patients with suspected cardiac etiology of arrest and ST elevation on ECG. When there is high suspicion of AMI, local protocols for treatment of AMI and coronary reperfusion should be activated. Coronary angiography, if indicated, can be beneficial in post–cardiac arrest patients regardless of whether they are awake or comatose. Even in the absence of ST elevation, emergent coronary angiography is reasonable for patients who are comatose after OHCA of suspected cardiac origin. Concurrent PCI and TTM are safe, with good outcomes reported for some comatose patients who have undergone PCI.

Critical care facilities that treat patients after cardiac arrest should use a comprehensive care plan that includes acute cardiovascular interventions, use of TTM, standardized medical goal-directed therapies, and advanced neurologic monitoring and care. Neurologic prognosis may be difficult to determine during the first 72 hours after resuscitation. This should be the earliest time to prognosticate a poor neurologic outcome in patients not treated with TTM. For those treated with TTM, providers should wait 72 hours after the patient returns to normothermia before prognosticating by using clinical examination where sedation or paralysis can be a confounder. Many initially comatose survivors of cardiac arrest have the potential for full recovery.[48,54,55] Therefore, it is important to place patients in a hospital critical care unit where expert care and neurologic evaluation can be performed and where appropriate testing to aid prognosis is performed in a timely manner.

Managing Post–Cardiac Arrest Care: The Post–Cardiac Arrest Care Algorithm

The Adult Immediate Post–Cardiac Arrest Care Algorithm (Figure 45) outlines all the steps for immediate assessment and management of post–cardiac arrest patients with ROSC. During this case, team members will continue to maintain good ventilation and oxygenation with a bag-mask device or advanced airway. Throughout the case discussion of the Post–Cardiac Arrest Care Algorithm, we will refer to Steps 1 through 8. These are the numbers assigned to the steps in the algorithm.

Use the H's and T's to recall conditions that could have contributed to the cardiac arrest. See column on the right of the algorithm and "Part 4: The Systematic Approach" for more information on the H's and T's, including clinical clues and suggested treatments.

Adult Immediate Post–Cardiac Arrest Care Algorithm—2015 Update

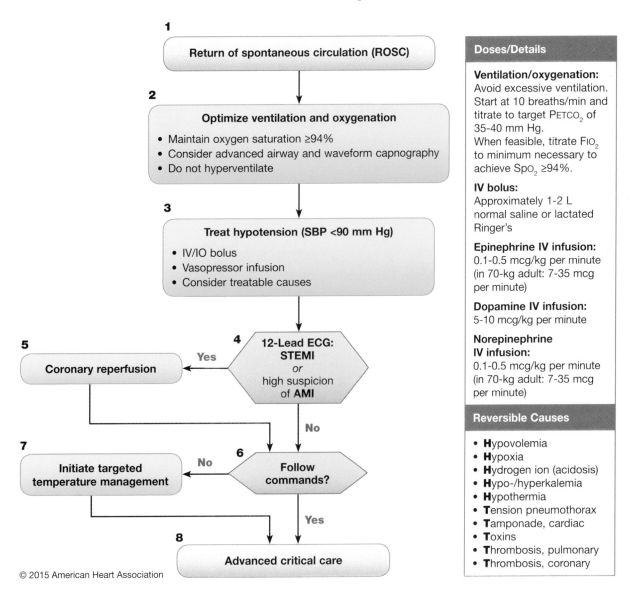

© 2015 American Heart Association

Figure 45. The Adult Immediate Post–Cardiac Arrest Care Algorithm.

Application of the Immediate Post–Cardiac Arrest Care Algorithm

Introduction

This case discusses the assessment and treatment of a patient who had cardiac arrest and was resuscitated with the use of the BLS Assessment and the ACLS Primary and Secondary Assessments. During rhythm check in the ACLS Primary Assessment, the patient's rhythm was organized and a pulse was detected (Step 12, Cardiac Arrest Algorithm [Figure 31]). The team leader will coordinate the efforts of the high-performance post–cardiac arrest care team as they perform the steps of the Post–Cardiac Arrest Care Algorithm.

Optimize Ventilation and Oxygenation

Step 2 directs you to ensure an adequate airway and support breathing immediately after ROSC. An unconscious/unresponsive patient will require an advanced airway for mechanical support of breathing.

- Use continuous waveform capnography to confirm and monitor correct placement of the ET tube (Figures 46 and 47).
- Use the lowest inspired oxygen concentration that will maintain arterial oxyhemoglobin saturation 94% or greater. When titration of inspired oxygen is not feasible (eg, in an out-of-hospital setting), it is reasonable to empirically use 100% oxygen until the patient arrives at the ED.
- Avoid excessive ventilation of the patient (do not ventilate too fast or too much). Providers may begin ventilations at 10/min and titrate to achieve a P_{ETCO_2} of 35 to 40 mm Hg or a $PaCO_2$ of 40 to 45 mm Hg.

To avoid hypoxia in adults with ROSC after cardiac arrest and if appropriate equipment is available, providers may use the highest available oxygen concentration until the arterial oxyhemoglobin saturation or the partial pressure of arterial oxygen can be measured. Decrease the fraction of inspired oxygen (FIO_2) when oxyhemoglobin saturation is 100%, provided the oxyhemoglobin saturation can be maintained for 94% or greater.

Because an oxygen saturation of 100% may correspond to a PaO_2 between approximately 80 and 500 mm Hg, in general it is appropriate to wean FIO_2 for a saturation of 100%, provided the patient can maintain oxyhemoglobin saturation of 94% or greater.

Critical Concepts

Waveform Capnography

In addition to monitoring ET tube position, quantitative waveform capnography allows healthcare personnel to monitor CPR quality, optimize chest compressions, and detect ROSC during chest compressions or when a rhythm check reveals an organized rhythm.

Caution

Things to Avoid During Ventilation

- When securing an advanced airway, avoid using ties that pass circumferentially around the patient's neck, thereby obstructing venous return from the brain.
- Excessive ventilation may potentially lead to adverse hemodynamic effects when intrathoracic pressures are increased and because of potential decreases in cerebral blood flow when $PaCO_2$ decreases.

Foundational Facts

Waveform Capnography

- End-tidal CO_2 is the concentration of carbon dioxide in exhaled air at the end of expiration. It is typically expressed as a partial pressure in millimeters of mercury (P_{ETCO_2}). Because CO_2 is a trace gas in atmospheric air, CO_2 detected by capnography in exhaled air is produced in the body and delivered to the lungs by circulating blood.
- Cardiac output is the major determinant of CO_2 delivery to the lungs. If ventilation is relatively constant, P_{ETCO_2} correlates well with cardiac output during CPR.
- Providers should observe a persistent capnographic waveform with ventilation to confirm and monitor ET tube placement in the field, in the transport vehicle, on arrival at the hospital, and after any patient transfer to reduce the risk of unrecognized tube misplacement or displacement.
- Although capnography to confirm and monitor correct placement of supraglottic airways (eg, laryngeal mask airway, laryngeal tube, or esophageal-tracheal tube) has not been studied, effective ventilation through a supraglottic airway device should result in a capnography waveform during CPR and after ROSC.

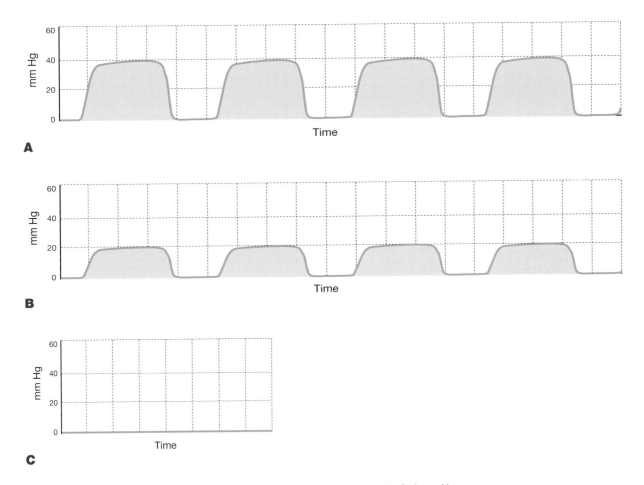

Figure 46. Waveform capnography. **A,** Normal range of 35 to 45 mm Hg. **B,** 20 mm Hg. **C,** 0 mm Hg.

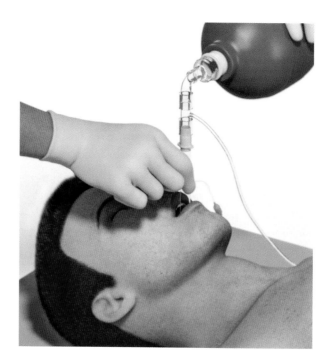

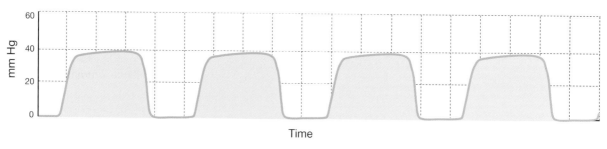

Time

Figure 47. Waveform capnography with an ET showing normal (adequate) ventilation pattern: PETCO₂ 35 to 40 mm Hg.

Treat Hypotension (SBP Less Than 90 mm Hg)

Box 3 directs you to treat hypotension when SBP is less than 90 mm Hg. Providers should obtain IV access if not already established. Verify the patency of any IV lines. ECG monitoring should continue after ROSC, during transport, and throughout ICU care until deemed clinically not necessary. At this stage, consider treating any reversible causes that might have precipitated the cardiac arrest but persist after ROSC.

When IV is established, treat hypotension as follows:

- **IV bolus** 1-2 L normal saline or lactated Ringer's
- **Norepinephrine** 0.1-0.5 mcg/kg per minute (in 70-kg adult: 7-35 mcg per minute) IV infusion titrated to achieve a minimum SBP of greater than 90 mm Hg or a mean arterial pressure of greater than 65 mm Hg
- **Epinephrine** 0.1-0.5 mcg/kg per minute (in 70-kg adult: 7-35 mcg per minute) IV infusion titrated to achieve a minimum SBP of greater than 90 mm Hg or a mean arterial pressure of greater than 65 mm Hg
- **Dopamine** 5-10 mcg/kg per minute IV infusion titrated to achieve a minimum SBP of greater than 90 mm Hg or a mean arterial pressure of greater than 65 mm Hg

Norepinephrine (levarterenol) is a naturally occurring potent vasoconstrictor and inotropic agent. It may be effective for management of patients with severe hypotension (eg, SBP less than 70 mm Hg) and a low total peripheral resistance who do not respond to less potent adrenergic drugs such as dopamine, phenylephrine, or methoxamine.

Epinephrine can be used in patients who are not in cardiac arrest but who require inotropic or vasopressor support.

Dopamine hydrochloride is a catecholamine-like agent and a chemical precursor of norepinephrine that stimulates the heart through both α- and β-adrenergic receptors.

STEMI Is Present or High Suspicion of AMI

Both in- and out-of-hospital medical personnel should obtain a 12-lead ECG as soon as possible after ROSC to identify those patients with STEMI or a high suspicion of AMI. Once such patients have been identified, hospital personnel should attempt coronary reperfusion (Step 5).

EMS personnel should transport these patients to a facility that reliably provides this therapy (Step 5).

Coronary Reperfusion

Aggressive treatment of STEMI, including coronary reperfusion with PCI, should begin if detected after ROSC, regardless of coma or TTM. In the case of out-of-hospital STEMI, provide advance notification to receiving facilities.

Following Commands

Step 4 directs you to examine the patient's ability to follow verbal commands.

If the patient does not follow commands, the high-performance team should consider implementing TTM (Step 7). If the patient is able to follow verbal commands, move to Step 8.

Targeted Temperature Management

To protect the brain and other organs, the high-performance team should start TTM in patients who remain comatose (lack of meaningful response to verbal commands) with ROSC after cardiac arrest.

For TTM, healthcare providers should select and maintain a constant target temperature between 32°C and 36°C for a period of at least 24 hours. Although the optimal method of achieving the target temperature is unknown, any combination of rapid infusion of ice-cold, isotonic, non–glucose-containing fluid (30 mL/kg), endovascular catheters, surface cooling devices, or simple surface interventions (eg, ice bags) appears to be safe and effective.

Specific features of the patient may favor selection of one temperature over another for TTM. Higher temperatures might be preferred in patients for whom lower temperatures convey some risk (eg, bleeding), and lower temperatures might be preferred when patients have clinical features that are worsened at higher temperatures (eg, seizures, cerebral edema). Of note, there are essentially no patients for whom temperature control somewhere in the range between 32°C and 36°C is contraindicated. Therefore, all patients in whom intensive care is continued are eligible.

In the prehospital setting, routine cooling of patients after ROSC with rapid infusion of cold IV fluids should not be done. Current evidence indicates that there is no direct outcome benefit from these interventions and that the IV fluid administration in the prehospital setting may increase pulmonary edema and rearrest. Whether different methods or devices for temperature control outside of the hospital are beneficial is unknown.

Foundational Facts

Targeted Temperature Management

- TTM is the only intervention demonstrated to improve neurologic recovery after cardiac arrest.
- The optimal duration of TTM is at least 24 hours. Comparative studies of the duration of TTM have not been performed in adults, but hypothermia for up to 72 hours was used safely in newborns.
- Healthcare providers should monitor the patient's core temperature during TTM by using an esophageal thermometer, bladder catheter in nonanuric patients, or a pulmonary artery catheter if one is placed for other indications. Axillary and oral temperatures are inadequate for measurement of core temperature changes.
- TTM should not affect the decision to perform PCI, because concurrent PCI and hypothermia are reported to be feasible and safe.

Advanced Critical Care

After coronary reperfusion interventions or in cases where the post–cardiac arrest patient has no ECG evidence or suspicion of MI, the high-performance team should transfer the patient to an ICU.

Post–Cardiac Arrest Maintenance Therapy

There is no evidence to support continued prophylactic administration of antiarrhythmic medications once the patient achieves ROSC.

Life Is Why

Science Is Why

Cardiovascular diseases claim more lives than all forms of cancer combined. This unsettling statistic drives the AHA's commitment to bring science to life by advancing resuscitation knowledge and research in new ways.

References

1. Jauch EC, Saver JL, Adams HP Jr, et al; American Heart Association Stroke Council, Council on Cardiovascular Nursing, Council on Peripheral Vascular Disease, Council on Clinical Cardiology. Guidelines for the early management of patients with acute ischemic stroke: a guideline for healthcare professionals from the American Heart Association/American Stroke Association. *Stroke.* 2013;44(3):870-947.

2. Adams HP Jr, del Zoppo G, Alberts MJ, et al; American Heart Association, American Stroke Association Stroke Council, Clinical Cardiology Council, Cardiovascular Radiology and Intervention Council, Atherosclerotic Peripheral Vascular Disease Quality of Care Outcomes in Research Interdisciplinary Working, Groups. Guidelines for the early management of adults with ischemic stroke: a guideline from the American Heart Association/American Stroke Association Stroke Council, Clinical Cardiology Council, Cardiovascular Radiology and Intervention Council, and the Atherosclerotic Peripheral Vascular Disease and Quality of Care Outcomes in Research Interdisciplinary Working Groups: the American Academy of Neurology affirms the value of this guideline as an educational tool for neurologists. *Stroke.* 2007;38(5):1655-1711.

3. Larsen MP, Eisenberg MS, Cummins RO, Hallstrom AP. Predicting survival from out-of-hospital cardiac arrest: a graphic model. *Ann Emerg Med.* 1993;22(11):1652-1658.

4. Valenzuela TD, Roe DJ, Cretin S, Spaite DW, Larsen MP. Estimating effectiveness of cardiac arrest interventions: a logistic regression survival model. *Circulation.* 1997;96(10):3308-3313.

5. Chan PS, Krumholz HM, Nichol G, Nallamothu BK. Delayed time to defibrillation after in-hospital cardiac arrest. *N Engl J Med.* 2008;358(1):9-17.

6. Stiell IG, Wells GA, Field B, et al. Advanced cardiac life support in out-of-hospital cardiac arrest. *N Engl J Med.* 2004;351(7):647-656.

7. Swor RA, Jackson RE, Cynar M, et al. Bystander CPR, ventricular fibrillation, and survival in witnessed, unmonitored out-of-hospital cardiac arrest. *Ann Emerg Med.* 1995;25(6):780-784.

8. Holmberg M, Holmberg S, Herlitz J. Incidence, duration and survival of ventricular fibrillation in out-of-hospital cardiac arrest patients in Sweden. *Resuscitation.* 2000;44(1):7-17.

9. Mentzelopoulos SD, Zakynthinos SG, Tzoufi M, et al. Vasopressin, epinephrine, and corticosteroids for in-hospital cardiac arrest. *Arch Intern Med.* 2009;169(1):15-24.

10. Mentzelopoulos SD, Malachias S, Chamos C, et al. Vasopressin, steroids, and epinephrine and neurologically favorable survival after in-hospital cardiac arrest: a randomized clinical trial. *JAMA.* 2013;310(3):270-279.

11. Paris PM, Stewart RD, Deggler F. Prehospital use of dexamethasone in pulseless idioventricular rhythm. *Ann Emerg Med.* 1984;13(11):1008-1010.

12. Tsai MS, Huang CH, Chang WT, et al. The effect of hydrocortisone on the outcome of out-of-hospital cardiac arrest patients: a pilot study. *Am J Emerg Med.* 2007;25(3):318-325.

13. Centers for Disease Control and Prevention. Injury prevention and control: prescription drug overdose. http://www.cdc.gov/drugoverdose/index.html. Accessed September 14, 2015.

14. Hedegaard H, Chen LH, Warner M. Drug-poisoning deaths involving heroin: United States, 2000–2013. http://www.cdc.gov/nchs/data/databriefs/db190.htm. Accessed September, 14, 2015.

15. Centers for Disease Control and Prevention. Fatal injury data. http://www.cdc.gov/injury/wisqars/fatal.html. Accessed September 14, 2015.

16. Carter CI, Graham B. Opioid overdose prevention and response in Canada. http://drugpolicy.ca/wp-content/uploads/2014/07CDPC_OverdosePreventionPolicy_Final_July2014.pdf. Accessed March 17, 2015.

17. Jones CM, Paulozzi LJ, Mack KA; Centers for Disease Control and Prevention (CDC). Alcohol involvement in opioid pain reliever and benzodiazepine drug abuse-related emergency department visits and drug-related deaths—United States, 2010. MMWR Morb Mortal Wkly Rep. 2014;63:881–885.

18. Madadi P, Hildebrandt D, Lauwers AE, Koren G. Characteristics of opioid-users whose death was related to opioid-toxicity: a population-based study in Ontario, Canada. *PLoS One.* 2013;8(4):e60600.

19. Webster LR, Cochella S, Dasgupta N, et al. An analysis of the root causes for opioid-related overdose deaths in the United States. *Pain Med.* 2011;12 Suppl 2:S26-35.

20. Paulozzi LJ, Logan JE, Hall AJ, McKinstry E, Kaplan JA, Crosby AE. A comparison of drug overdose deaths involving methadone and other opioid analgesics in West Virginia. *Addiction.* 2009;104(9):1541-1548.

21. Krantz MJ, Kutinsky IB, Robertson AD, Mehler PS. Dose-related effects of methadone on QT prolongation in a series of patients with torsade de pointes. *Pharmacotherapy.* 2003;23(6):802-805.

22. Eap CB, Crettol S, Rougier JS, et al. Stereoselective block of hERG channel by (S)-methadone and QT interval prolongation in CYP2B6 slow metabolizers. *Clin Pharmacol Ther.* 2007;81(5):719-728.

23. Krantz MJ, Martin J, Stimmel B, Mehta D, Haigney MC. QTc interval screening in methadone treatment. *Ann Intern Med.* 2009;150(6):387-395.

24. Stallvik M, Nordstrand B, Kristensen O, Bathen J, Skogvoll E, Spigset O. Corrected QT interval during treatment with methadone and buprenorphine—relation to doses and serum concentrations. *Drug Alcohol Depend.* 2013;129(1-2):88-93.

25. Chou R, Weimer MB, Dana T. Methadone overdose and cardiac arrhythmia potential: findings from a review of the evidence for an American Pain Society and College on Problems of Drug Dependence clinical practice guideline. *J Pain.* 2014;15(4):338-365.

26. Lipski J, Stimmel B, Donoso E. The effect of heroin and multiple drug abuse on the electrocardiogram. *Am Heart J.* 1973;86(5):663-668.

27. Labi M. Paroxysmal atrial fibrillation in heroin intoxication. *Ann Intern Med.* 1969;71(5):951-959.

28. Leach M. Naloxone: a new therapeutic and diagnostic agent for emergency use. *J Amer Coll Emerg Phys.* 1973;2:21-23.

29. Sporer KA, Firestone J, Isaacs SM. Out-of-hospital treatment of opioid overdoses in an urban setting. *Acad Emerg Med.* 1996;3(7):660-667.

30. Robertson TM, Hendey GW, Stroh G, Shalit M. Intranasal naloxone is a viable alternative to intravenous naloxone for prehospital narcotic overdose. *Prehosp Emerg Care.* 2009;13(4):512-515.

31. Evans LE, Swainson CP, Roscoe P, Prescott LF. Treatment of drug overdosage with naloxone, a specific narcotic antagonist. *Lancet.* 1973;1(7801):452-455.

32. Kelly AM, Kerr D, Dietze P, Patrick I, Walker T, Koutsogiannis Z. Randomised trial of intranasal versus intramuscular naloxone in prehospital treatment for suspected opioid overdose. *Med J Aust.* 2005;182(1):24-27.

33. Barton ED, Colwell CB, Wolfe T, et al. Efficacy of intranasal naloxone as a needleless alternative for treatment of opioid overdose in the prehospital setting. *J Emerg Med.* 2005;29(3):265-271.

34. Wolfe TR, Braude DA. Intranasal medication delivery for children: a brief review and update. *Pediatrics.* 2010;126(3):532-537.

35. Loimer N, Hofmann P, Chaudhry HR. Nasal administration of naloxone is as effective as the intravenous route in opiate addicts. *Int J Addict.* 1994;29(6):819-827.

36. Doe-Simkins M, Walley AY, Epstein A, Moyer P. Saved by the nose: bystander-administered intranasal naloxone hydrochloride for opioid overdose. *Am J Public Health.* 2009;99(5):788-791.

37. Wanger K, Brough L, Macmillan I, Goulding J, MacPhail I, Christenson JM. Intravenous vs subcutaneous naloxone for out-of-hospital management of presumed opioid overdose. *Acad Emerg Med.* 1998;5(4):293-299.

38. Baumann BM, Patterson RA, Parone DA, et al. Use and efficacy of nebulized naloxone in patients with suspected opioid intoxication. *Am J Emerg Med.* 2013;31(3):585-588.

39. Weber JM, Tataris KL, Hoffman JD, Aks SE, Mycyk MB. Can nebulized naloxone be used safely and effectively by emergency medical services for suspected opioid overdose? *Prehosp Emerg Care.* 2012;16(2):289-292.

40. Greenberg MI, Roberts JR, Baskin SI. Endotracheal naloxone reversal of morphine-induced respiratory depression in rabbits. *Ann Emerg Med.* 1980;9(6):289-292.

41. Callaway CW, Schmicker R, Kampmeyer M, et al. Receiving hospital characteristics associated with survival after out-of-hospital cardiac arrest. *Resuscitation.* 2010;81(5):524-529.

42. Carr BG, Kahn JM, Merchant RM, Kramer AA, Neumar RW. Inter-hospital variability in post-cardiac arrest mortality. *Resuscitation.* 2009;80(1):30-34.

43. Laurent I, Monchi M, Chiche JD, et al. Reversible myocardial dysfunction in survivors of out-of-hospital cardiac arrest. *J Am Coll Cardiol.* 2002;40(12):2110-2116.

44. Negovsky VA. The second step in resuscitation—the treatment of the "post-resuscitation disease." *Resuscitation.* 1972;1(1):1-7.

45. Safar P. Resuscitation from clinical death: pathophysiologic limits and therapeutic potentials. *Crit Care Med.* 1988;16(10):923-941.

46. Neumar RW, Nolan JP, Adrie C, et al. Post-cardiac arrest syndrome: epidemiology, pathophysiology, treatment, and prognostication. A consensus statement from the International Liaison Committee on Resuscitation (American Heart Association, Australian and New Zealand Council on Resuscitation, European Resuscitation Council, Heart and Stroke Foundation of Canada, InterAmerican Heart Foundation, Resuscitation Council of Asia, and the Resuscitation Council of Southern Africa); the American Heart Association Emergency Cardiovascular Care Committee; the Council on Cardiovascular Surgery and Anesthesia; the Council on Cardiopulmonary, Perioperative, and Critical Care; the Council on Clinical Cardiology; and the Stroke Council. *Circulation.* 2008;118(23):2452-2483.

47. Skrifvars MB, Pettila V, Rosenberg PH, Castren M. A multiple logistic regression analysis of in-hospital factors related to survival at six months in patients resuscitated from out-of-hospital ventricular fibrillation. *Resuscitation.* 2003;59(3):319-328.

48. Gaieski DF, Band RA, Abella BS, et al. Early goal-directed hemodynamic optimization combined with therapeutic hypothermia in comatose survivors of out-of-hospital cardiac arrest. *Resuscitation.* 2009;80(4):418-424.

49. Sunde K, Pytte M, Jacobsen D, et al. Implementation of a standardised treatment protocol for post resuscitation care after out-of-hospital cardiac arrest. *Resuscitation.* 2007;73(1):29-39.

50. Kirves H, Skrifvars MB, Vahakuopus M, Ekstrom K, Martikainen M, Castren M. Adherence to resuscitation guidelines during prehospital care of cardiac arrest patients. *Eur J Emerg Med.* 2007;14(2):75-81.

51. Laver S, Farrow C, Turner D, Nolan J. Mode of death after admission to an intensive care unit following cardiac arrest. *Intensive Care Med.* 2004;30(11):2126-2128.

52. Anyfantakis ZA, Baron G, Aubry P, et al. Acute coronary angiographic findings in survivors of out-of-hospital cardiac arrest. *Am Heart J.* 2009;157(2):312-318.

53. Spaulding CM, Joly LM, Rosenberg A, et al. Immediate coronary angiography in survivors of out-of-hospital cardiac arrest. *N Engl J Med.* 1997;336(23):1629-1633.

54. Bunch TJ, White RD, Gersh BJ, et al. Long-term outcomes of out-of-hospital cardiac arrest after successful early defibrillation. *N Engl J Med.* 2003;348(26):2626-2633.

55. Hypothermia After Cardiac Arrest Study Group. Mild therapeutic hypothermia to improve the neurologic outcome after cardiac arrest. *N Engl J Med.* 2002;346(8):549-556.

Appendix

Adult High-Quality BLS
Skills Testing Checklist

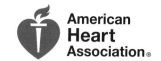

American **Heart** Association®

life is why™

Student Name _____ Date of Test _____

Hospital Scenario: "You are working in a hospital or clinic, and you see a person who has suddenly collapsed in the hallway. You check that the scene is safe and then approach the patient. Demonstrate what you would do next."

Prehospital Scenario: "You arrive on the scene for a suspected cardiac arrest. No bystander CPR has been provided. You approach the scene and ensure that it is safe. Demonstrate what you would do next."

Assessment and Activation
☐ Checks responsiveness   ☐ Shouts for help/Activates emergency response system/Sends for AED
☐ Checks breathing   ☐ Checks pulse

Once student shouts for help, instructor says, "Here's the barrier device. I am going to get the AED."

Cycle 1 of CPR (30:2)   **CPR feedback devices preferred for accuracy*

Adult Compressions
☐ Performs high-quality compressions*:
- Hand placement on lower half of sternum
- 30 compressions in no less than 15 and no more than 18 seconds
- Compresses at least 2 inches (5 cm)
- Complete recoil after each compression

Adult Breaths
☐ Gives 2 breaths with a barrier device:
- Each breath given over 1 second
- Visible chest rise with each breath
- Resumes compressions in less than 10 seconds

Cycle 2 of CPR (repeats steps in Cycle 1)   *Only check box if step is successfully performed*
☐ Compressions   ☐ Breaths   ☐ Resumes compressions in less than 10 seconds

Rescuer 2 says, "Here is the AED. I'll take over compressions, and you use the AED."

AED (follows prompts of AED)
☐ Powers on AED   ☐ Correctly attaches pads   ☐ Clears for analysis   ☐ Clears to safely deliver a shock
☐ Safely delivers a shock

Resumes Compressions
☐ Ensures compressions are resumed immediately after shock delivery
- Student directs instructor to resume compressions *or*
- Second student resumes compressions

STOP TEST

Instructor Notes
- Place a ✓ in the box next to each step the student completes successfully.
- If the student does not complete all steps successfully (as indicated by at least 1 blank check box), the student must receive remediation. Make a note here of which skills require remediation (refer to Instructor Manual for information about remediation).

Test Results	Circle **PASS** or **NR** to indicate pass or needs remediation:	**PASS**	**NR**

Instructor Initials _____ Instructor Number _____ Date _____

Airway Management Skills Testing Checklist

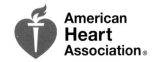

Student Name _____ Date of Test _____

Critical Performance Steps	✓ if done correctly
BLS Assessment and Interventions	
Checks for responsiveness • Taps and shouts, "Are you OK?"	
Activates the emergency response system • Shouts for nearby help/Activates the emergency response system and gets the AED *or* • Directs second rescuer to activate the emergency response system and get the AED	
Checks breathing • Scans chest for movement (5-10 seconds)	
Checks pulse (5-10 seconds) **Breathing and pulse check can be done simultaneously** Notes that pulse is present and does not initiate chest compressions or attach AED	
Inserts oropharyngeal or nasopharyngeal airway	
Administers oxygen	
Performs effective bag-mask ventilation for 1 minute • Gives proper ventilation rate (once every 5-6 seconds) • Gives proper ventilation speed (over 1 second) • Gives proper ventilation volume (~half a bag)	

STOP TEST

Test Results	Circle **PASS** or **NR** to indicate pass or needs remediation:	**PASS**	**NR**

Instructor Initials _____ Instructor Number _____ Date _____

Instructor Notes
- Place a ✓ in the box next to each step the student completes successfully.
- If the student does not complete all steps successfully (as indicated by at least 1 blank check box), the student must receive remediation. Make a note here of which skills require remediation (refer to Instructor Manual for information about remediation).

Test Results	Circle **PASS** or **NR** to indicate pass or needs remediation:	**PASS**	**NR**

Instructor Initials _____ Instructor Number _____ Date _____

Megacode Testing Checklist: Scenarios 1/3/8
Bradycardia → Pulseless VT → PEA → PCAC

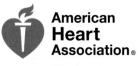

American Heart Association®

life is why™

Student Name _____ Date of Test _____

Critical Performance Steps	✓ if done correctly
Team Leader	
Ensures high-quality CPR at all times	
Assigns team member roles	
Ensures that team members perform well	
Bradycardia Management	
Starts oxygen if needed, places monitor, starts IV	
Places monitor leads in proper position	
Recognizes symptomatic bradycardia	
Administers correct dose of atropine	
Prepares for second-line treatment	
Pulseless VT Management	
Recognizes pVT	
Clears before analyze and shock	
Immediately resumes CPR after shocks	
Appropriate airway management	
Appropriate cycles of drug–rhythm check/shock–CPR	
Administers appropriate drug(s) and doses	
PEA Management	
Recognizes PEA	
Verbalizes potential reversible causes of PEA (H's and T's)	
Administers appropriate drug(s) and doses	
Immediately resumes CPR after rhythm checks	
Post–Cardiac Arrest Care	
Identifies ROSC	
Ensures BP and 12-lead ECG are performed, O_2 saturation is monitored, verbalizes need for endotracheal intubation and waveform capnography, and orders laboratory tests	
Considers targeted temperature management	

STOP TEST

Test Results	Circle **PASS** or **NR** to indicate pass or needs remediation:	**PASS**	**NR**

Instructor Initials _____ Instructor Number _____ Date _____

Learning Station Competency

☐ Cardiac Arrest ☐ Bradycardia ☐ Tachycardia ☐ Immediate Post–Cardiac Arrest Care ☐ Megacode Practice

Megacode Testing Checklist: Scenarios 2/5
Bradycardia → VF → Asystole → PCAC

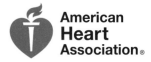

Student Name _____ Date of Test _____

Critical Performance Steps	✓ if done correctly
Team Leader	
Ensures high-quality CPR at all times	
Assigns team member roles	
Ensures that team members perform well	
Bradycardia Management	
Starts oxygen if needed, places monitor, starts IV	
Places monitor leads in proper position	
Recognizes symptomatic bradycardia	
Administers correct dose of atropine	
Prepares for second-line treatment	
VF Management	
Recognizes VF	
Clears before analyze and shock	
Immediately resumes CPR after shocks	
Appropriate airway management	
Appropriate cycles of drug–rhythm check/shock–CPR	
Administers appropriate drug(s) and doses	
Asystole Management	
Recognizes asystole	
Verbalizes potential reversible causes of asystole (H's and T's)	
Administers appropriate drug(s) and doses	
Immediately resumes CPR after rhythm checks	
Post–Cardiac Arrest Care	
Identifies ROSC	
Ensures BP and 12-lead ECG are performed, O$_2$ saturation is monitored, verbalizes need for endotracheal intubation and waveform capnography, and orders laboratory tests	
Considers targeted temperature management	

STOP TEST

Test Results	Circle **PASS** or **NR** to indicate pass or needs remediation:	PASS	NR

Instructor Initials _____ Instructor Number _____ Date _____

Learning Station Competency

☐ Cardiac Arrest ☐ Bradycardia ☐ Tachycardia ☐ Immediate Post–Cardiac Arrest Care ☐ Megacode Practice

Megacode Testing Checklist: Scenarios 4/7/10
Tachycardia → VF → PEA → PCAC

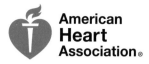

Student Name _____ Date of Test _____

Critical Performance Steps	✓ if done correctly
Team Leader	
Ensures high-quality CPR at all times	
Assigns team member roles	
Ensures that team members perform well	
Tachycardia Management	
Starts oxygen if needed, places monitor, starts IV	
Places monitor leads in proper position	
Recognizes unstable tachycardia	
Recognizes symptoms due to tachycardia	
Performs immediate synchronized cardioversion	
VF Management	
Recognizes VF	
Clears before analyze and shock	
Immediately resumes CPR after shocks	
Appropriate airway management	
Appropriate cycles of drug–rhythm check/shock–CPR	
Administers appropriate drug(s) and doses	
PEA Management	
Recognizes PEA	
Verbalizes potential reversible causes of PEA (H's and T's)	
Administers appropriate drug(s) and doses	
Immediately resumes CPR after rhythm checks	
Post–Cardiac Arrest Care	
Identifies ROSC	
Ensures BP and 12-lead ECG are performed, O₂ saturation is monitored, verbalizes need for endotracheal intubation and waveform capnography, and orders laboratory tests	
Considers targeted temperature management	

STOP TEST

Test Results	Circle **PASS** or **NR** to indicate pass or needs remediation:	**PASS**	**NR**
Instructor Initials _____ Instructor Number _____ Date _____			

Learning Station Competency

☐ Cardiac Arrest ☐ Bradycardia ☐ Tachycardia ☐ Immediate Post–Cardiac Arrest Care ☐ Megacode Practice

Megacode Testing Checklist: Scenarios 6/11
Bradycardia → VF → PEA → PCAC

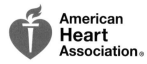

American
Heart
Association®

life is why™

Student Name _____ Date of Test _____

Critical Performance Steps	✓ if done correctly
Team Leader	
Ensures high-quality CPR at all times	
Assigns team member roles	
Ensures that team members perform well	
Bradycardia Management	
Starts oxygen if needed, places monitor, starts IV	
Places monitor leads in proper position	
Recognizes symptomatic bradycardia	
Administers correct dose of atropine	
Prepares for second-line treatment	
VF Management	
Recognizes VF	
Clears before analyze and shock	
Immediately resumes CPR after shocks	
Appropriate airway management	
Appropriate cycles of drug–rhythm check/shock–CPR	
Administers appropriate drug(s) and doses	
PEA Management	
Recognizes PEA	
Verbalizes potential reversible causes of PEA (H's and T's)	
Administers appropriate drug(s) and doses	
Immediately resumes CPR after rhythm checks	
Post–Cardiac Arrest Care	
Identifies ROSC	
Ensures BP and 12-lead ECG are performed, O$_2$ saturation is monitored, verbalizes need for endotracheal intubation and waveform capnography, and orders laboratory tests	
Considers targeted temperature management	

STOP TEST

Test Results	Circle **PASS** or **NR** to indicate pass or needs remediation:	PASS	NR
Instructor Initials _____ Instructor Number _____ Date _____			

Learning Station Competency

☐ Cardiac Arrest ☐ Bradycardia ☐ Tachycardia ☐ Immediate Post–Cardiac Arrest Care ☐ Megacode Practice

© 2016 American Heart Association

Megacode Testing Checklist: Scenario 9
Tachycardia → PEA → VF → PCAC

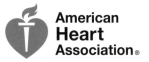
American Heart Association®
life is why™

Student Name _____ Date of Test _____

Critical Performance Steps	✓ if done correctly
Team Leader	
Ensures high-quality CPR at all times	
Assigns team member roles	
Ensures that team members perform well	
Tachycardia Management	
Starts oxygen if needed, places monitor, starts IV	
Places monitor leads in proper position	
Recognizes tachycardia (specific diagnosis)	
Recognizes no symptoms due to tachycardia	
Considers appropriate initial drug therapy	
PEA Management	
Recognizes PEA	
Verbalizes potential reversible causes of PEA (H's and T's)	
Administers appropriate drug(s) and doses	
Immediately resumes CPR after rhythm check and pulse checks	
VF Management	
Recognizes VF	
Clears before analyze and shock	
Immediately resumes CPR after shocks	
Appropriate airway management	
Appropriate cycles of drug–rhythm check/shock–CPR	
Administers appropriate drug(s) and doses	
Post–Cardiac Arrest Care	
Identifies ROSC	
Ensures BP and 12-lead ECG are performed, O$_2$ saturation is monitored, verbalizes need for endotracheal intubation and waveform capnography, and orders laboratory tests	
Considers targeted temperature management	

STOP TEST

Test Results	Circle **PASS** or **NR** to indicate pass or needs remediation:	**PASS**	**NR**
Instructor Initials _____	Instructor Number _____	Date _____	

Learning Station Competency

☐ Cardiac Arrest ☐ Bradycardia ☐ Tachycardia ☐ Immediate Post–Cardiac Arrest Care ☐ Megacode Practice

Megacode Testing Checklist: Scenario 12
Bradycardia → VF → Asystole/PEA → PCAC

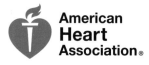

American **Heart** Association®

life is why™

Student Name _____ Date of Test _____

Critical Performance Steps	✓ if done correctly
Team Leader	
Ensures high-quality CPR at all times	
Assigns team member roles	
Ensures that team members perform well	
Bradycardia Management	
Starts oxygen if needed, places monitor, starts IV	
Places monitor leads in proper position	
Recognizes symptomatic bradycardia	
Administers correct dose of atropine	
Prepares for second-line treatment	
VF Management	
Recognizes VF	
Clears before analyze and shock	
Immediately resumes CPR after shocks	
Appropriate airway management	
Appropriate cycles of drug–rhythm check/shock–CPR	
Administers appropriate drug(s) and doses	
Asystole and PEA Management	
Recognizes asystole and PEA	
Verbalizes potential reversible causes of asystole and PEA (H's and T's)	
Administers appropriate drug(s) and doses	
Immediately resumes CPR after rhythm checks	
Post–Cardiac Arrest Care	
Identifies ROSC	
Ensures BP and 12-lead ECG are performed, O_2 saturation is monitored, verbalizes need for endotracheal intubation and waveform capnography, and orders laboratory tests	
Considers targeted temperature management	

STOP TEST

Test Results	Circle **PASS** or **NR** to indicate pass or needs remediation:	**PASS**	**NR**
Instructor Initials _____	Instructor Number _____	Date _____	

Learning Station Competency

☐ Cardiac Arrest ☐ Bradycardia ☐ Tachycardia ☐ Immediate Post–Cardiac Arrest Care ☐ Megacode Practice

© 2016 American Heart Association

Cardiac Arrest VF/Pulseless VT Learning Station Checklist

Adult Cardiac Arrest Algorithm—2015 Update

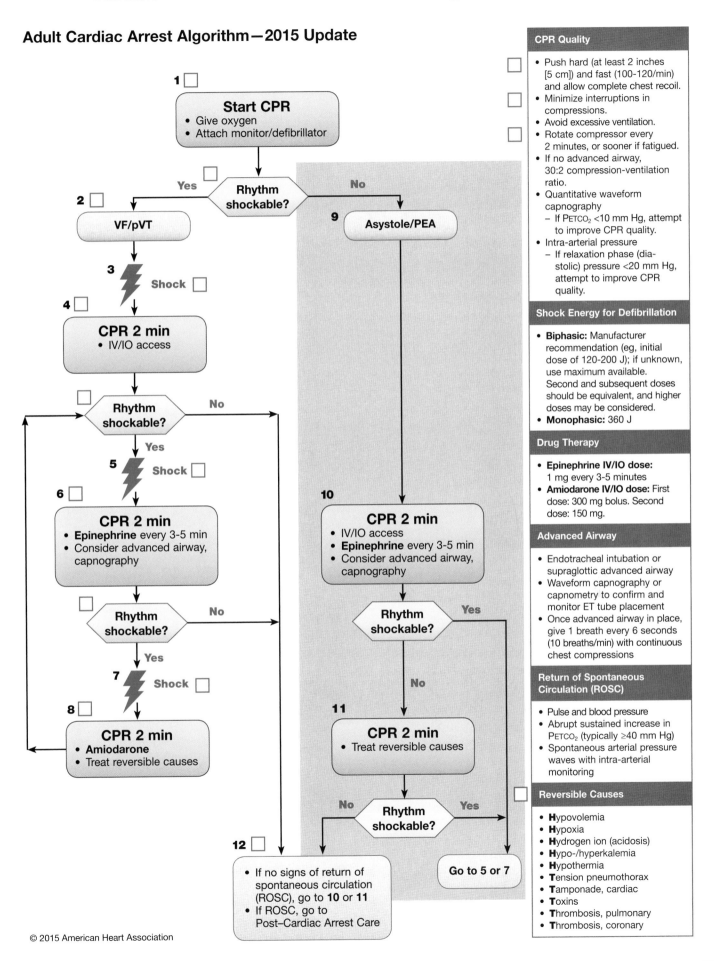

CPR Quality

- Push hard (at least 2 inches [5 cm]) and fast (100-120/min) and allow complete chest recoil.
- Minimize interruptions in compressions.
- Avoid excessive ventilation.
- Rotate compressor every 2 minutes, or sooner if fatigued.
- If no advanced airway, 30:2 compression-ventilation ratio.
- Quantitative waveform capnography
  - If P_{ETCO_2} <10 mm Hg, attempt to improve CPR quality.
- Intra-arterial pressure
  - If relaxation phase (diastolic) pressure <20 mm Hg, attempt to improve CPR quality.

Shock Energy for Defibrillation

- **Biphasic:** Manufacturer recommendation (eg, initial dose of 120-200 J); if unknown, use maximum available. Second and subsequent doses should be equivalent, and higher doses may be considered.
- **Monophasic:** 360 J

Drug Therapy

- **Epinephrine IV/IO dose:** 1 mg every 3-5 minutes
- **Amiodarone IV/IO dose:** First dose: 300 mg bolus. Second dose: 150 mg.

Advanced Airway

- Endotracheal intubation or supraglottic advanced airway
- Waveform capnography or capnometry to confirm and monitor ET tube placement
- Once advanced airway in place, give 1 breath every 6 seconds (10 breaths/min) with continuous chest compressions

Return of Spontaneous Circulation (ROSC)

- Pulse and blood pressure
- Abrupt sustained increase in P_{ETCO_2} (typically ≥40 mm Hg)
- Spontaneous arterial pressure waves with intra-arterial monitoring

Reversible Causes

- **H**ypovolemia
- **H**ypoxia
- **H**ydrogen ion (acidosis)
- **H**ypo-/hyperkalemia
- **H**ypothermia
- **T**ension pneumothorax
- **T**amponade, cardiac
- **T**oxins
- **T**hrombosis, pulmonary
- **T**hrombosis, coronary

Cardiac Arrest Asystole/PEA Learning Station Checklist

Adult Cardiac Arrest Algorithm—2015 Update

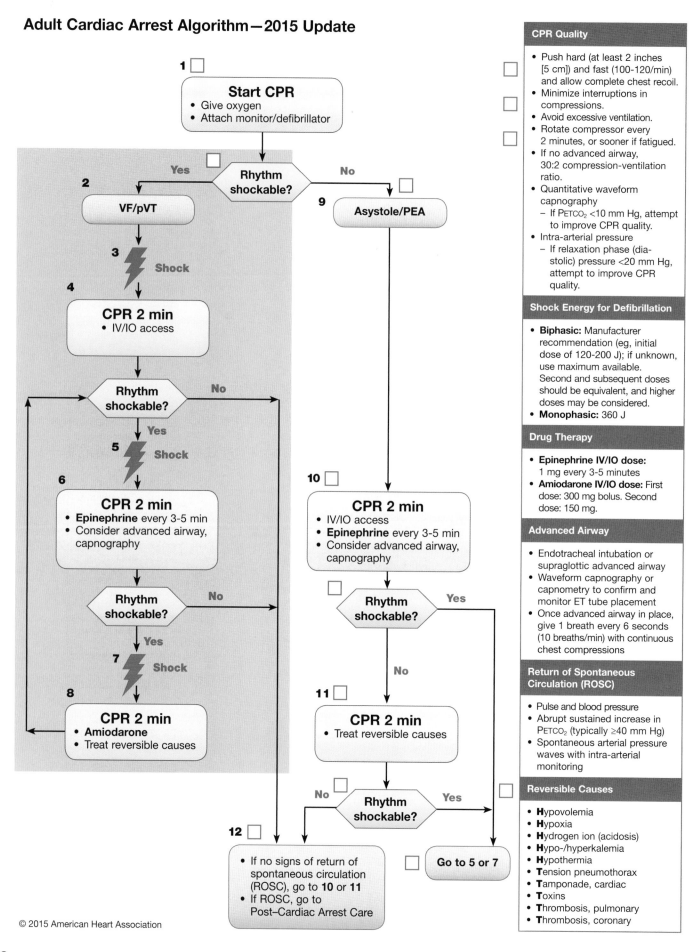

1 ☐

Start CPR
- Give oxygen
- Attach monitor/defibrillator

☐ **Rhythm shockable?**

Yes → **2** VF/pVT

No → **9** ☐ Asystole/PEA

3 Shock

4

CPR 2 min
- IV/IO access

Rhythm shockable? — **No**

Yes — **5** Shock

6

CPR 2 min
- **Epinephrine** every 3-5 min
- Consider advanced airway, capnography

Rhythm shockable? — **No**

Yes — **7** Shock

8

CPR 2 min
- **Amiodarone**
- Treat reversible causes

10 ☐

CPR 2 min
- IV/IO access
- **Epinephrine** every 3-5 min
- Consider advanced airway, capnography

☐ **Rhythm shockable?** — **Yes**

No

11 ☐

CPR 2 min
- Treat reversible causes

☐ **Rhythm shockable?** — **Yes** ☐ **Go to 5 or 7**

No

12 ☐
- If no signs of return of spontaneous circulation (ROSC), go to **10** or **11**
- If ROSC, go to Post–Cardiac Arrest Care

CPR Quality
☐
- Push hard (at least 2 inches [5 cm]) and fast (100-120/min) and allow complete chest recoil.
☐
- Minimize interruptions in compressions.
- Avoid excessive ventilation.
☐
- Rotate compressor every 2 minutes, or sooner if fatigued.
- If no advanced airway, 30:2 compression-ventilation ratio.
- Quantitative waveform capnography
  - If P_{ETCO_2} <10 mm Hg, attempt to improve CPR quality.
- Intra-arterial pressure
  - If relaxation phase (diastolic) pressure <20 mm Hg, attempt to improve CPR quality.

Shock Energy for Defibrillation
- **Biphasic:** Manufacturer recommendation (eg, initial dose of 120-200 J); if unknown, use maximum available. Second and subsequent doses should be equivalent, and higher doses may be considered.
- **Monophasic:** 360 J

Drug Therapy
- **Epinephrine IV/IO dose:** 1 mg every 3-5 minutes
- **Amiodarone IV/IO dose:** First dose: 300 mg bolus. Second dose: 150 mg.

Advanced Airway
- Endotracheal intubation or supraglottic advanced airway
- Waveform capnography or capnometry to confirm and monitor ET tube placement
- Once advanced airway in place, give 1 breath every 6 seconds (10 breaths/min) with continuous chest compressions

Return of Spontaneous Circulation (ROSC)
- Pulse and blood pressure
- Abrupt sustained increase in P_{ETCO_2} (typically ≥40 mm Hg)
- Spontaneous arterial pressure waves with intra-arterial monitoring

Reversible Causes
- **H**ypovolemia
- **H**ypoxia
- **H**ydrogen ion (acidosis)
- **H**ypo-/hyperkalemia
- **H**ypothermia
- **T**ension pneumothorax
- **T**amponade, cardiac
- **T**oxins
- **T**hrombosis, pulmonary
- **T**hrombosis, coronary

Bradycardia Learning Station Checklist

Adult Bradycardia With a Pulse Algorithm

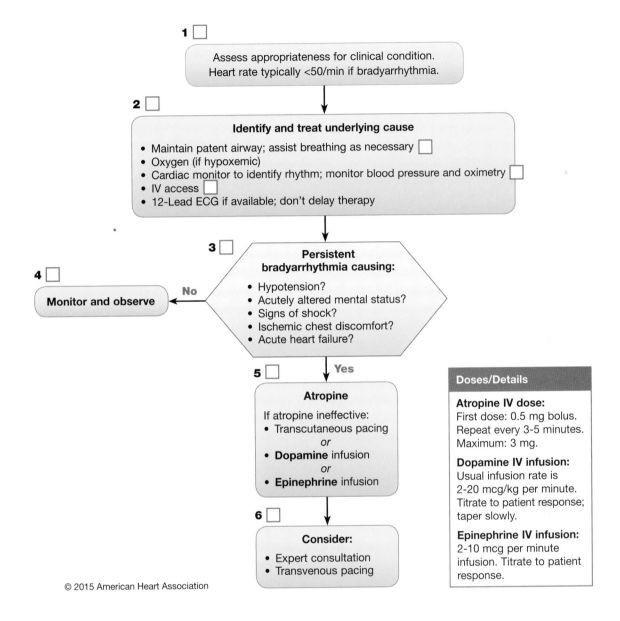

1 ☐ Assess appropriateness for clinical condition. Heart rate typically <50/min if bradyarrhythmia.

2 ☐ **Identify and treat underlying cause**
- Maintain patent airway; assist breathing as necessary ☐
- Oxygen (if hypoxemic)
- Cardiac monitor to identify rhythm; monitor blood pressure and oximetry ☐
- IV access ☐
- 12-Lead ECG if available; don't delay therapy

3 ☐ **Persistent bradyarrhythmia causing:**
- Hypotension?
- Acutely altered mental status?
- Signs of shock?
- Ischemic chest discomfort?
- Acute heart failure?

4 ☐ **Monitor and observe** ← **No**

Yes

5 ☐ **Atropine**

If atropine ineffective:
- Transcutaneous pacing
  or
- **Dopamine** infusion
  or
- **Epinephrine** infusion

6 ☐ **Consider:**
- Expert consultation
- Transvenous pacing

Doses/Details

Atropine IV dose:
First dose: 0.5 mg bolus.
Repeat every 3-5 minutes.
Maximum: 3 mg.

Dopamine IV infusion:
Usual infusion rate is
2-20 mcg/kg per minute.
Titrate to patient response;
taper slowly.

Epinephrine IV infusion:
2-10 mcg per minute
infusion. Titrate to patient
response.

Tachycardia Learning Station Checklist

Adult Tachycardia With a Pulse Algorithm

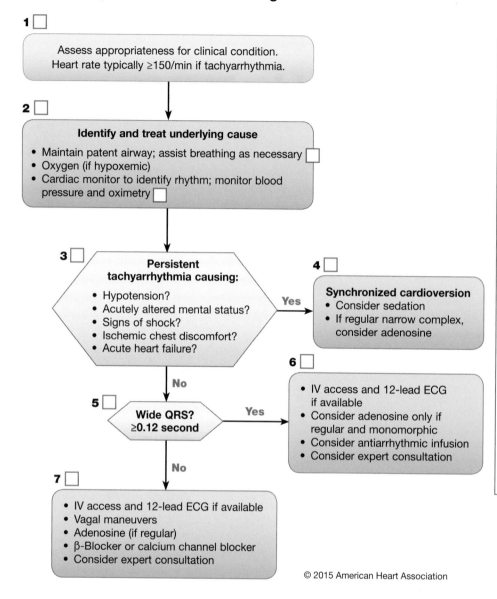

1 ☐

Assess appropriateness for clinical condition.
Heart rate typically ≥150/min if tachyarrhythmia.

2 ☐

Identify and treat underlying cause

- Maintain patent airway; assist breathing as necessary ☐
- Oxygen (if hypoxemic)
- Cardiac monitor to identify rhythm; monitor blood pressure and oximetry ☐

3 ☐

Persistent tachyarrhythmia causing:

- Hypotension?
- Acutely altered mental status?
- Signs of shock?
- Ischemic chest discomfort?
- Acute heart failure?

Yes →

4 ☐

Synchronized cardioversion

- Consider sedation
- If regular narrow complex, consider adenosine

No

5 ☐

Wide QRS?
≥0.12 second

Yes →

6 ☐

- IV access and 12-lead ECG if available
- Consider adenosine only if regular and monomorphic
- Consider antiarrhythmic infusion
- Consider expert consultation

No

7 ☐

- IV access and 12-lead ECG if available
- Vagal maneuvers
- Adenosine (if regular)
- β-Blocker or calcium channel blocker
- Consider expert consultation

© 2015 American Heart Association

Doses/Details

Synchronized cardioversion:
Initial recommended doses:
- Narrow regular: 50-100 J
- Narrow irregular: 120-200 J biphasic or 200 J monophasic
- Wide regular: 100 J
- Wide irregular: defibrillation dose (*not* synchronized)

Adenosine IV dose:
First dose: 6 mg rapid IV push; follow with NS flush.
Second dose: 12 mg if required.

Antiarrhythmic Infusions for Stable Wide-QRS Tachycardia

Procainamide IV dose:
20-50 mg/min until arrhythmia suppressed, hypotension ensues, QRS duration increases >50%, or maximum dose 17 mg/kg given. Maintenance infusion: 1-4 mg/min. Avoid if prolonged QT or CHF.

Amiodarone IV dose:
First dose: 150 mg over 10 minutes. Repeat as needed if VT recurs. Follow by maintenance infusion of 1 mg/min for first 6 hours.

Sotalol IV dose:
100 mg (1.5 mg/kg) over 5 minutes. Avoid if prolonged QT.

Immediate Post–Cardiac Arrest Care Learning Station Checklist

Adult Immediate Post–Cardiac Arrest Care Algorithm—2015 Update

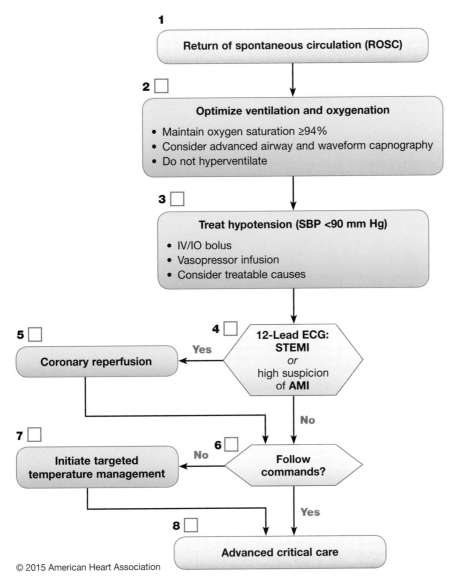

1
Return of spontaneous circulation (ROSC)

2 ☐
Optimize ventilation and oxygenation
- Maintain oxygen saturation ≥94%
- Consider advanced airway and waveform capnography
- Do not hyperventilate

3 ☐
Treat hypotension (SBP <90 mm Hg)
- IV/IO bolus
- Vasopressor infusion
- Consider treatable causes

4 ☐
12-Lead ECG: STEMI *or* high suspicion of **AMI**

5 ☐ ← Yes
Coronary reperfusion

6 ☐
Follow commands?

7 ☐ ← No
Initiate targeted temperature management

No →

Yes ↓

8 ☐
Advanced critical care

© 2015 American Heart Association

Doses/Details

Ventilation/oxygenation:
Avoid excessive ventilation. Start at 10 breaths/min and titrate to target P_{ETCO_2} of 35-40 mm Hg.
When feasible, titrate F_{IO_2} to minimum necessary to achieve SpO_2 ≥94%.

IV bolus:
Approximately 1-2 L
normal saline or lactated Ringer's

Epinephrine IV infusion:
0.1-0.5 mcg/kg per minute (in 70-kg adult: 7-35 mcg per minute)

Dopamine IV infusion:
5-10 mcg/kg per minute

Norepinephrine IV infusion:
0.1-0.5 mcg/kg per minute (in 70-kg adult: 7-35 mcg per minute)

☐ **Reversible Causes**

- **H**ypovolemia
- **H**ypoxia
- **H**ydrogen ion (acidosis)
- **H**ypo-/hyperkalemia
- **H**ypothermia
- **T**ension pneumothorax
- **T**amponade, cardiac
- **T**oxins
- **T**hrombosis, pulmonary
- **T**hrombosis, coronary

ACLS Pharmacology Summary Table

Drug	Indications	Precautions/Contraindications	Adult Dosage
Adenosine	• First drug for most forms of stable narrow-complex SVT. Effective in terminating those due to reentry involving AV node or sinus node • May consider for unstable narrow-complex reentry tachycardia while preparations are made for cardioversion • Regular and monomorphic wide-complex tachycardia, thought to be or previously defined to be reentry SVT • Does *not* convert atrial fibrillation, atrial flutter, or VT • Diagnostic maneuver: stable narrow-complex SVT	• Contraindicated in poison/drug-induced tachycardia or second- or third-degree heart block • Transient side effects include flushing, chest pain or tightness, brief periods of asystole or bradycardia, ventricular ectopy • Less effective (larger doses may be required) in patients taking theophylline or caffeine • Reduce initial dose to 3 mg in patients receiving dipyridamole or carbamazepine, in heart transplant patients, or if given by central venous access • If administered for irregular, polymorphic wide-complex tachycardia/VT, may cause deterioration (including hypotension) • Transient periods of sinus bradycardia and ventricular ectopy are common after termination of SVT • Safe and effective in pregnancy	**IV Rapid Push** • Place patient in mild reverse Trendelenburg position before administration of drug • Initial bolus of 6 mg given rapidly over 1 to 3 seconds followed by NS bolus of 20 mL; then elevate the extremity • A second dose (12 mg) can be given in 1 to 2 minutes if needed **Injection Technique** • Record rhythm strip during administration • Draw up adenosine dose and flush in 2 separate syringes • Attach both syringes to the IV injection port closest to patient • Clamp IV tubing above injection port • Push IV adenosine as quickly as possible (1 to 3 seconds) • While maintaining pressure on adenosine plunger, push NS flush as rapidly as possible after adenosine • Unclamp IV tubing
Amiodarone	Because its use is associated with toxicity, amiodarone is indicated for use in patients with life-threatening arrhythmias when administered with appropriate monitoring: • VF/pulseless VT unresponsive to shock delivery, CPR, and a vasopressor • Recurrent, hemodynamically unstable VT *With expert consultation,* amiodarone may be used for treatment of some atrial and ventricular arrhythmias	*Caution:* **Multiple complex drug interactions** • Rapid infusion may lead to hypotension • With multiple dosing, cumulative doses >2.2 g over 24 hours are associated with significant hypotension in clinical trials • Do not administer with other drugs that prolong QT interval (eg, procainamide) • Terminal elimination is extremely long (half-life lasts up to 40 days)	**VF/pVT Cardiac Arrest Unresponsive to CPR, Shock, and Vasopressor** • **First dose:** 300 mg IV/IO push • **Second dose (if needed):** 150 mg IV/IO push **Life-Threatening Arrhythmias** **Maximum cumulative dose:** 2.2 g IV over 24 hours. May be administered as follows: • **Rapid infusion:** 150 mg IV over first 10 minutes (15 mg per minute). May repeat rapid infusion (150 mg IV) every 10 minutes as needed • **Slow infusion:** 360 mg IV over 6 hours (1 mg per minute) • **Maintenance infusion:** 540 mg IV over 18 hours (0.5 mg per minute)

(continued)

Drug	Indications	Precautions/ Contraindications	Adult Dosage
Atropine Sulfate *Can be given via endotracheal tube*	• First drug for symptomatic sinus bradycardia • May be beneficial in presence of AV nodal block. **Not likely to be effective for type II second-degree or third-degree AV block or a block in nonnodal tissue** • Routine use during PEA or asystole is unlikely to have a therapeutic benefit • Organophosphate (eg, nerve agent) poisoning: extremely large doses may be needed	• Use with caution in presence of myocardial ischemia and hypoxia. Increases myocardial oxygen demand • Avoid in hypothermic bradycardia • May not be effective for infranodal (type II) AV block and new third-degree block with wide QRS complexes. (In these patients, may cause paradoxical slowing. Be prepared to pace or give catecholamines) • Doses of atropine <0.5 mg may result in paradoxical slowing of heart rate	**Bradycardia (With or Without ACS)** • 0.5 mg IV every 3 to 5 minutes as needed, not to exceed total dose of 0.04 mg/kg (total 3 mg) • Use shorter dosing interval (3 minutes) and higher doses in severe clinical conditions **Organophosphate Poisoning** Extremely large doses (2 to 4 mg or higher) may be needed
Dopamine *IV infusion*	• Second-line drug for symptomatic bradycardia (after atropine) • Use for hypotension (SBP ≤70 to 100 mm Hg) with signs and symptoms of shock	• Correct hypovolemia with volume replacement before initiating dopamine • Use with caution in cardiogenic shock with accompanying CHF • May cause tachyarrhythmias, excessive vasoconstriction • Do not mix with sodium bicarbonate	**IV Administration** • Usual infusion rate is 2 to 20 mcg/kg per minute • Titrate to patient response; taper slowly
Epinephrine *Can be given via endotracheal tube* *Available in 1:10 000 and 1:1000 concentrations*	• **Cardiac arrest:** VF, pulseless VT, asystole, PEA • **Symptomatic bradycardia:** Can be considered after atropine as an alternative infusion to dopamine • **Severe hypotension:** Can be used when pacing and atropine fail, when hypotension accompanies bradycardia, or with phosphodiesterase enzyme inhibitor • **Anaphylaxis, severe allergic reactions:** Combine with large fluid volume, corticosteroids, antihistamines	• Raising blood pressure and increasing heart rate may cause myocardial ischemia, angina, and increased myocardial oxygen demand • High doses do not improve survival or neurologic outcome and may contribute to postresuscitation myocardial dysfunction • Higher doses may be required to treat poison/drug-induced shock	**Cardiac Arrest** • **IV/IO dose:** 1 mg (10 mL of 1:10 000 solution) administered every 3 to 5 minutes during resuscitation. Follow each dose with 20 mL flush, elevate arm for 10 to 20 seconds after dose • **Higher dose:** Higher doses (up to 0.2 mg/kg) may be used for specific indications (β-blocker or calcium channel blocker overdose) • **Continuous infusion:** Initial rate: 0.1 to 0.5 mcg/kg per minute (for 70-kg patient: 7 to 35 mcg per minute); titrate to response • **Endotracheal route:** 2 to 2.5 mg diluted in 10 mL NS **Profound Bradycardia or Hypotension** 2 to 10 mcg per minute infusion; titrate to patient response

(continued)

Drug	Indications	Precautions/Contraindications	Adult Dosage
Lidocaine *Can be given via endotracheal tube*	• Alternative to amiodarone in cardiac arrest from VF/pVT • Stable monomorphic VT with preserved ventricular function • Stable polymorphic VT with normal baseline QT interval and preserved LV function when ischemia is treated and electrolyte balance is corrected • Can be used for stable polymorphic VT with baseline • QT-interval prolongation if torsades suspected	• **Contraindication:** Prophylactic use in AMI is contraindicated • Reduce maintenance dose (not loading dose) in presence of impaired liver function or LV dysfunction • Discontinue infusion immediately if signs of toxicity develop	**Cardiac Arrest From VF/pVT** • Initial dose: 1 to 1.5 mg/kg IV/IO • For refractory VF, may give additional 0.5 to 0.75 mg/kg IV push, repeat in 5 to 10 minutes; maximum 3 doses or total of 3 mg/kg **Perfusing Arrhythmia** For stable VT, wide-complex tachycardia of uncertain type, significant ectopy: • Doses ranging from 0.5 to 0.75 mg/kg and up to 1 to 1.5 mg/kg may be used • Repeat 0.5 to 0.75 mg/kg every 5 to 10 minutes; maximum total dose: 3 mg/kg **Maintenance Infusion** 1 to 4 mg per minute (30 to 50 mcg/kg per minute)
Magnesium Sulfate	• Recommended for use in cardiac arrest only if torsades de pointes or suspected hypomagnesemia is present • Life-threatening ventricular arrhythmias due to digitalis toxicity • Routine administration in hospitalized patients with AMI is not recommended	• Occasional fall in blood pressure with rapid administration • Use with caution if renal failure is present	**Cardiac Arrest (Due to Hypomagnesemia or Torsades de Pointes)** 1 to 2 g (2 to 4 mL of a 50% solution diluted in 10 mL [eg, D_5W, normal saline] given IV/IO) **Torsades de Pointes With a Pulse or AMI With Hypomagnesemia** • Loading dose of 1 to 2 g mixed in 50 to 100 mL of diluent (eg, D_5W, normal saline) over 5 to 60 minutes IV • Follow with 0.5 to 1 g per hour IV (titrate to control torsades)

2015 Science Summary Table

Topic	2010	2015

Systematic Approach: BLS Assessment (name change)	• 1-2-3-4
	• Check responsiveness:
	  – Tap and shout
	  – Scan chest for movement
	• Activate the emergency response system and get an AED
	• Circulation: Check the carotid pulse. If you cannot detect a pulse within 10 seconds, start CPR, beginning with chest compressions, immediately
	• Defibrillation: If indicated, deliver a shock with an AED or defibrillator
		• Check responsiveness
		  – Tap and shout
		• Shout for nearby help/activate emergency response system/get AED
		• Check breathing and pulse (simultaneously)
		• Defibrillation: If indicated, deliver a shock with an AED or defibrillator

Systematic Approach: Primary Assessment (name change)	• Airway • Breathing • Circulation • Differential diagnosis (H's and T's)	• Airway • Breathing • Circulation • Disability • Exposure
Systematic Approach: Secondary Assessment (new)	• NA	• SAMPLE • H's and T's
BLS: High-Quality CPR	• A rate of at least 100 chest compressions per minute • A compression depth of at least 2 inches in adults • Allowing complete chest recoil after each compression • Minimizing interruptions in compressions (10 seconds or less) • Avoiding excessive ventilation • Switching providers about every 2 minutes to avoid fatigue	• A rate of 100 to 120 chest compressions per minute • A compression depth of at least 2 inches in adults* • Allowing complete chest recoil after each compression • Minimizing interruptions in compressions (10 seconds or less) • Avoiding excessive ventilation • Chest compression fraction of at least 60% but ideally greater than 80% • Switch compressor about every 2 minutes or sooner if fatigued • Use of audio and visual feedback devices to monitor CPR quality *When a feedback device is available, adjust to a maximum depth of 2.4 inches [6 cm]) in adolescents and adults.

(continued)

(continued)

Topic	2010	2015
ACLS: Immediate Post–Cardiac Arrest Care	• Consider therapeutic hypothermia (32°C to 34°C for 12 to 24 hours) to optimize survival and neurologic recovery in comatose patients	• Consider targeted temperature management to optimize survival and neurologic recovery in comatose patients—cool to 32°C to 36°C for at least 24 hours • Out-of-hospital cooling of patients with rapid infusion of cold IV fluids after ROSC is not recommended
ACLS: Managing the Airway	• For cardiac arrest with an advanced airway in place, ventilate once every 6 to 8 seconds	• For cardiac arrest with an advanced airway in place, ventilate once every 6 seconds
ACLS: Bradycardia	• Dopamine dosing: 2 to 10 mcg/kg per minute	• Dopamine dosing: 2 to 20 mcg/kg per minute
ACLS: ACS	• NSTEMI • Titrate O$_2$ saturation to ≥94%	• NSTE-ACS • Titrate O$_2$ saturation to ≥90%

Topic	2015
ACLS: Cardiac Arrest	• Removed vasopressin from the Cardiac Arrest Algorithm • Administer epinephrine as soon as feasible after the onset of cardiac arrest due to an initial nonshockable rhythm • Added Opioid-Associated Life-Threatening Emergency (Adult) Algorithm • Healthcare providers tailor the sequence of rescue actions based on the presumed etiology of the arrest. Moreover, ACLS providers functioning within a high-performance team can choose the optimal approach for minimizing interruptions in chest compressions (thereby improving chest compression fraction [CCF]). Use of different protocols, such as 3 cycles of 200 continuous compressions with passive oxygen insufflation and airway adjuncts, compression-only CPR in the first few minutes after arrest, and continuous chest compressions with asynchronous ventilation once every 6 seconds with the use of a bag-mask device, are a few examples of optimizing CCF and high-quality CPR. A default compression-to-ventilation ratio of 30:2 should be used by less-trained healthcare providers or if 30:2 is the established protocol. • Consider using ultrasound during arrest to detect underlying causes (eg, PE) • Extracorporeal CPR may be considered among select cardiac arrest patients who have not responded to initial conventional CPR, in settings where it can be rapidly implemented • Consider administering intravenous lipid emulsion, concomitant with standard resuscitative care, to patients who have premonitory neurotoxicity or cardiac arrest due to local anesthetic toxicity or other forms of drug toxicity and who are failing standard resuscitative measures
ACLS: Stroke	• Endovascular therapy (treatment window up to 6 hours)

Glossary

A	
Acute	Having a sudden onset and short course
Acute myocardial infarction (AMI)	The early critical stage of necrosis of heart muscle tissue caused by blockage of a coronary artery
Advanced cardiovascular life support (ACLS)	Emergency medical procedures in which basic life support efforts of CPR are supplemented with drug administration, IV fluids, etc
Asystole	Absence of electrical and mechanical activity in the heart
Atrial fibrillation	In atrial fibrillation the atria "quiver" chaotically and the ventricles beat irregularly
Atrial flutter	Rapid, irregular atrial contractions due to an abnormality of atrial excitation
Atrioventricular (AV) block	A delay in the normal flow of electrical impulses that cause the heart to beat
Automated external defibrillator (AED)	A portable device used to restart a heart that has stopped

B	
Basic life support (BLS)	Emergency treatment of a victim of cardiac or respiratory arrest through cardiopulmonary resuscitation and emergency cardiovascular care
Bradycardia	Slow heartbeat, whether physiologically or pathologically

C	
Capnography	The measurement and graphic display of CO_2 levels in the airways, which can be performed by infrared spectroscopy
Cardiac arrest	Temporary or permanent cessation of the heartbeat
Cardiopulmonary resuscitation (CPR)	A basic emergency procedure for life support, consisting of mainly manual external cardiac massage and some artificial respiration
Coronary syndrome	A group of clinical symptoms compatible with acute myocardial ischemia. Also called *coronary heart disease.*
Coronary thrombosis	The blocking of the coronary artery of the heart by a thrombus

E	
Electrocardiogram (ECG)	A test that provides a typical record of normal heart action
Endotracheal (ET) intubation	The passage of a tube through the nose or mouth into the trachea for maintenance of the airway
Esophageal-tracheal tube	A double-lumen tube with inflatable balloon cuffs that seal off the hypopharynx from the oropharynx and esophagus; used for airway management

H	
Hydrogen ion (acidosis)	The accumulation of acid and hydrogen ions or depletion of the alkaline reserve (bicarbonate content) in the blood and body tissues, decreasing the pH
Hyperkalemia	An abnormally high concentration of potassium ions in the blood. Also called *hyperpotassemia.*
Hypoglycemia	An abnormally low concentration of glucose in the blood
Hypokalemia	An abnormally low concentration of potassium ions in the blood. Also called *hypopotassemia.*
Hypothermia	A potentially fatal condition that occurs when body temperature falls below 95°F (35°C)
Hypovolemia	A decrease in the volume of circulating blood
Hypoxia	A deficiency of oxygen reaching the tissues of the body

I	
Intraosseous (IO)	Within a bone
Intravenous (IV)	Within a vein
M	
Mild hypothermia	When the patient's body temperature is between 90°F and 95°F
Moderate hypothermia	When the patient's body temperature is between 86°F and 93.2°F
N	
Nasopharyngeal	Pertaining to the nose and pharynx
O	
Oropharyngeal airway	A tube used to provide free passage of air between the mouth and pharynx
P	
Perfusion	The passage of fluid (such as blood) through a specific organ or area of the body (such as the heart)
Prophylaxis	Prevention of or protection against disease
Pulmonary edema (PE)	A condition in which fluid accumulates in the lungs
Pulseless electrical activity (PEA)	Continued electrical rhythmicity of the heart in the absence of effective mechanical function
R	
Recombinant tissue plasminogen activator (rtPA)	A clot-dissolving substance produced naturally by cells in the walls of blood vessels
S	
Severe hypothermia	When the patient's body temperature is <86°F
Sinus rhythm	The rhythm of the heart produced by impulses from the sinoatrial node
Supraglottic	Situated or occurring above the glottis
Synchronized cardioversion	Uses a sensor to deliver a shock that is synchronized with a peak in the QRS complex
Syncope	A loss of consciousness over a short period of time, caused by a temporary lack of oxygen in the brain
T	
Tachycardia	Increased heartbeat, usually ≥100/min
Tamponade (cardiac)	A condition caused by accumulation of fluid between the heart and the pericardium, resulting in excess pressure on the heart. This impairs the heart's ability to pump sufficient blood.
Tension pneumothorax	Pneumothorax resulting from a wound in the chest wall which acts as a valve that permits air to enter the pleural cavity but prevents its escape
Thrombus	A blood clot formed within a blood vessel
U	
Unsynchronized shock	An electrical shock that will be delivered as soon as the operator pushes the shock button to discharge the defibrillator. Thus, the shock can fall anywhere within the cardiac cycle.
V	
Ventricular fibrillation (VF)	Very rapid uncoordinated fluttering contractions of the ventricles
Ventricular tachycardia (VT)	A rapid heartbeat that originates in one of the lower chambers (ventricles) of the heart

Foundation Index

Index